Rachel Pauls, M.D., knows it is vital for optimal gut health to move through the reintroduction phase of the low-FODMAP diet. Her book, *The FODMAP Reintroduction Plan & Cookbook*, steers you through this most complex process, as she has IBS herself. This book shows you how to reintroduce foods and which foods to choose. It explains when you have "passed" a food challenge and provides Pauls' original, family-friendly recipes that use the new foods that you will be introducing. The low-FODMAP diet is ultimately about eating as broadly as possible without triggering your IBS symptoms. **This book will help you achieve success.**

> **—Dédé Wilson, co-founder of FODMAP Everyday® and author of *The Low-FODMAP Diet Step-by-Step***

The most challenging part of the low-FODMAP diet is the second phase, where patients reintroduce foods containing FODMAPs to determine their sensitivities. Dr. Rachel Pauls's new book provides a guided tour through the reintroduction phase. For doctors, *The FODMAP Reintroduction Plan & Cookbook* provides a medically responsible way to help patients find their own version of the low-FODMAP diet. For dietitians, it is a reliable way to reinforce the concepts they review. For patients, this book provides an easy-to-read and beautifully illustrated atlas to navigate the low-FODMAP diet. **We will be adding *The FODMAP Reintroduction Plan & Cookbook* to our resources for patients.**

> **—William D. Chey, M.D., AGAF, FACG, FACP, RFF, H. Marvin Pollard Professor of Gastroenterology, Professor of Nutrition Sciences, Chief, Division of Gastroenterology, University of Michigan**

Rachel Pauls, M.D., provides practical and actionable steps for the often-overlooked reintroduction phase of the low-FODMAP diet. She empowers you with a **clear plan and innovative recipes to help you figure out your food triggers with ease!**

> **—Katelyn Wilson, R.D., IBS, and digestive health specialist, expert in integrative and functional nutrition, www.HealthyGutFx.com**

This book will help IBS patients who have had a good symptom response to the low-FODMAP diet take necessary steps to pinpoint their FODMAP symptom triggers. Dr. Rachel Pauls **guides readers through thirteen FODMAP reintroductions and provides wise advice on how to interpret the results.** Because there is less research specifically about the reintroduction phase, it is hard to find credible information about how it should be done. Dr. Pauls fills that void in a book that is clearly written, well organized, and consistent with expert opinion.

> **—Patsy Catsos, M.S., RDN, LD, expert gastroenterology dietitian, medical nutrition therapist and author of *The IBS Elimination Diet and Cookbook, IBS-Free at Last, and the IBS-Free FODMAP Toolkit for RDNs*, www.ibsfree.net**

THE
FODMAP
Reintroduction
PLAN & COOKBOOK

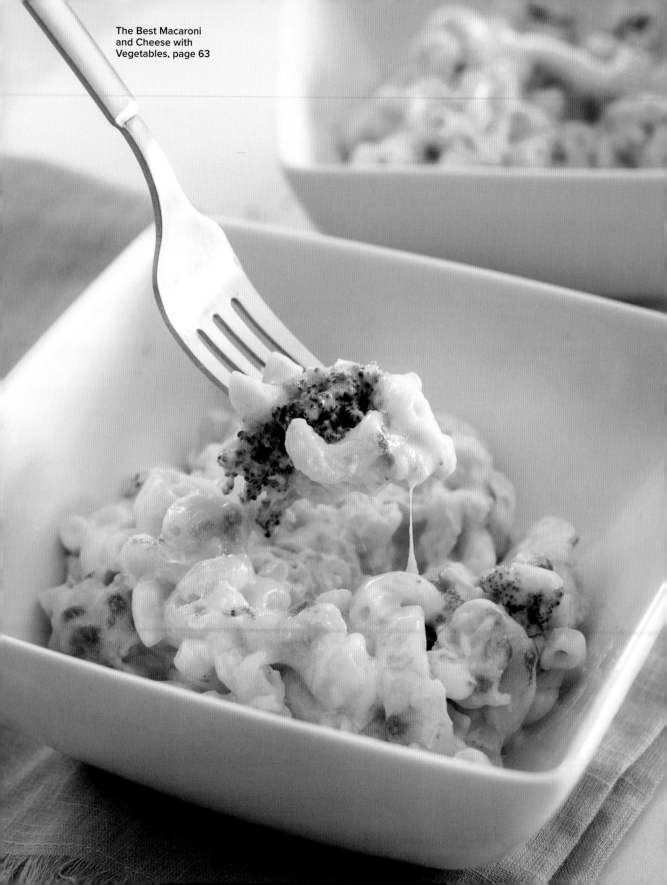

The Best Macaroni
and Cheese with
Vegetables, page 63

THE
FODMAP
Reintroduction
PLAN & COOKBOOK

Conquer Your IBS While Reclaiming the Foods You Love

Rachel Pauls, M.D.

FAIR WINDS

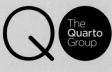

Inspiring | Educating | Creating | Entertaining

Brimming with creative inspiration, how-to projects, and useful information to enrich your everyday life, quarto.com is a favorite destination for those pursuing their interests and passions.

First Published in 2023 by Fair Winds Press, an imprint of The Quarto Group,
100 Cummings Center, Suite 265-D, Beverly, MA 01915, USA.
T (978) 282-9590 F (978) 283-2742 Quarto.com

Fair Winds Press titles are also available at discount for retail, wholesale, promotional, and bulk purchase. For details, contact the Special Sales Manager by email at specialsales@quarto.com or by mail at The Quarto Group, Attn: Special Sales Manager, 100 Cummings Center, Suite 265-D, Beverly, MA 01915, USA.

27 26 25 24 23   1 2 3 4 5

ISBN: 978-0-7603-8275-2

Digital edition published in 2023
eISBN: 978-0-7603-8276-9

Design: John Hall Design Group, Beverly, MA
Photography: Alison Bickel
Illustration: Rachel Pauls Food

Printed in China

Library of Congress Cataloging-in-Publication Data

Pauls, Rachel, author.

The FODMAP reintroduction plan and cookbook : conquer your IBS while reclaiming the foods you love /

Rachel Pauls, M.D. Beverly, MA : Fair Winds Press, an imprint of the Quarto Group, 2023. | Includes index. | LCCN 2022049420 (print) | LCCN 2022049421 (ebook) | ISBN 9780760382752 (paperback) | ISBN 9780760382769 (ebook)

AN IMPORTANT NOTE FROM DR. PAULS:

This book should not be relied upon for medical or dietary advice or replace the care of a health care provider. The research and science surrounding FODMAPs and IBS are rapidly evolving. While the recipes in this book are intended to be low-FODMAP based upon available information at the time of writing (2022), none of them has been subjected to formal laboratory analysis for FODMAPs. If you experience negative symptoms related to any of the recipes, stop eating that food and contact your health care provider.

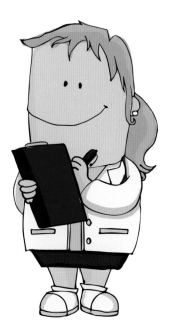

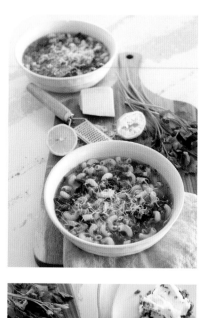
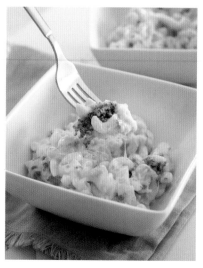
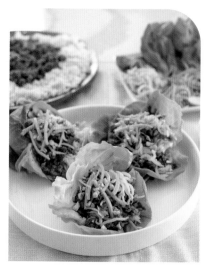
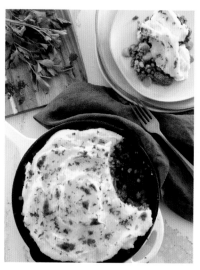
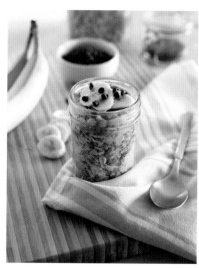
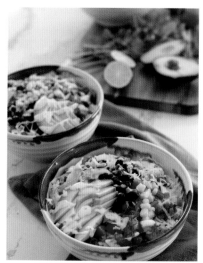
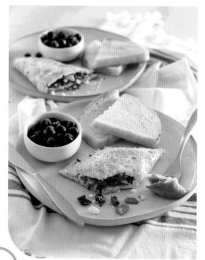
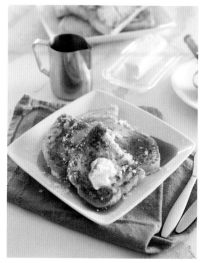
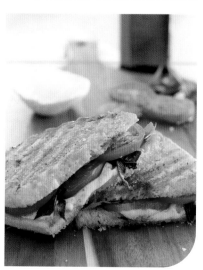

CONTENTS

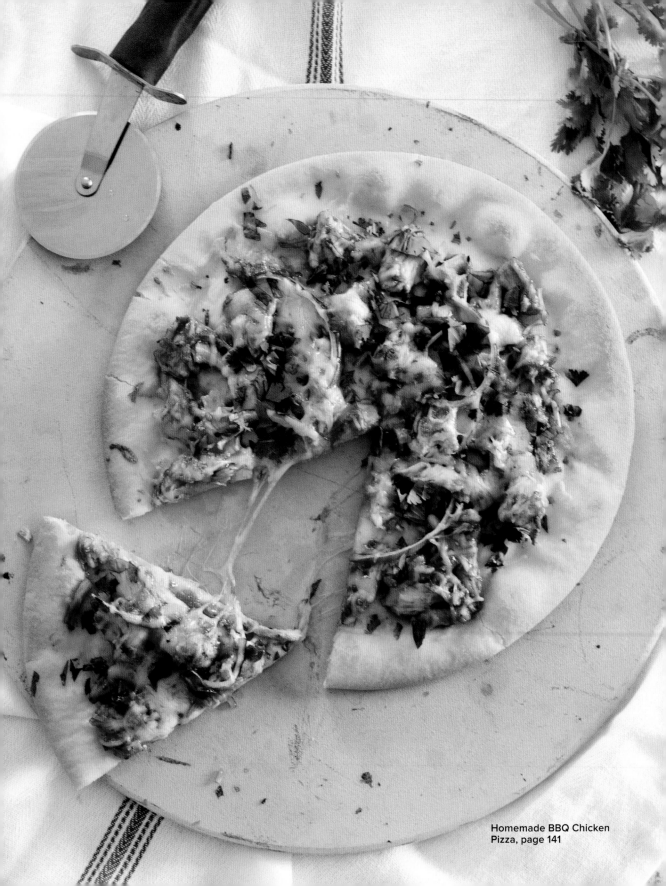

Homemade BBQ Chicken
Pizza, page 141

INTRODUCTION

Hello friends,

Welcome to this exciting new chapter of healing your IBS. My book is going to take you through the second phase of the low-FODMAP diet: **reintroduction**. (This is also known as the *FODMAP Challenge Phase*.)

During this phase, you will carefully add foods back to your diet, with the aim of building an understanding of *which FODMAPs you can tolerate*. Reintroduction enhances your food options, meal flexibility, *and* digestive balance.

Completing these important steps will get you closer to your final goal: **personalization**. I will provide guidance on this final phase of the low-FODMAP diet as well, in the last chapter of this book.

Until today, you have been learning and living the elimination phase of the low-FODMAP diet. Your IBS symptoms are under control, which is AMAZING. But you're probably wondering, what comes next? How, and when, can you get back to normal life?

I know *exactly* how you feel. Reintroduction is a mysterious and intimidating process. There's little information out there to guide you, and you may be nervous about triggering your IBS. That's the main reason I wrote this book: to provide you the help you need.

First, an important disclaimer: This book does not replace the advice of a dietitian. If you have the means to work with someone during this phase, then I absolutely endorse that option. However, if it's not a possibility in your life, my book will guide and support you.

For those of you who haven't met me, let me give you some background on my story. I have been a medical doctor and educator for twenty-five years. As a board-certified specialist in female pelvic medicine and reconstructive surgery (urogynecology), I have cared for thousands of women and have intricate knowledge of the pelvic anatomy. I counsel patients daily about their GI symptoms and believe strongly in the role diet plays in improving quality of life. I am a researcher with more than a hundred publications, including papers on the low-FODMAP diet. My acclaimed first book, *The Low-FODMAP*

IBS Solution Plan and Cookbook, has successfully helped thousands of people begin the path toward digestive wellness.

But there is more. Like you, I have IBS. And I have been where you are.

A low-FODMAP diet healed my body *and my life* several years ago. Once I felt better, I didn't know how to advance in my low-FODMAP journey. So, I learned all about reintroduction, then guided myself through it. I made mistakes and gained valuable lessons. Now I will be sharing my knowledge with you.

I will walk you through this next phase, one step at a time. In section I, we'll discuss the basic principles of the FODMAP diet, and the rationale behind reintroduction. I will teach you the different types of FODMAPs, and how to gently test each one to learn how you react to it. I will provide suggestions and strategies, and thirty-eight unique low-FODMAP recipes to support your body during testing. Then, in section II, we will cover the thirteen FODMAP reintroduction categories and their recommended test foods. This section includes twenty-two customized recipes to use for the challenges, along with detailed portion sizes and more tips and tricks. Finally, I will review integration and personalization, the final phase of your modified low-FODMAP lifestyle.

This book has everything you need to succeed.

You will conquer reintroduction on your own terms. No rush. No deadlines. My goal is to keep you feeling your absolute best. Who has time to flare? I don't, and neither do you.

By the end of this book, you will have discovered which FODMAPs you can tolerate, and in what amounts. You will have more freedom in your cooking, eating, and living. It won't be easy, but it *will* be worth it.

Are you ready to start learning about this amazing new chapter in your IBS and FODMAP journey?

Let's do this. Together.

Rachel Pauls

Rachel Pauls, M.D.

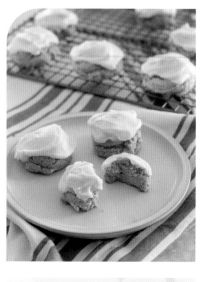
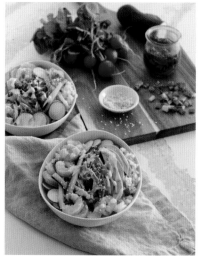
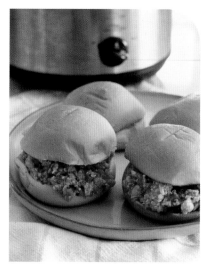
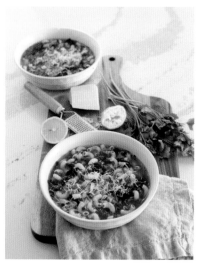
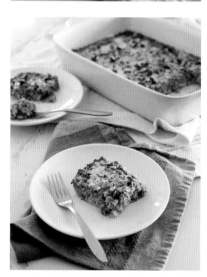
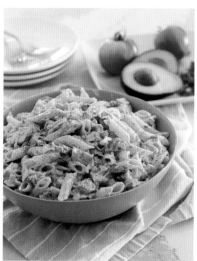
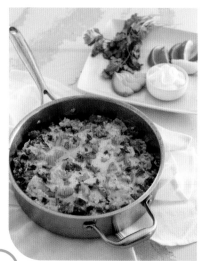
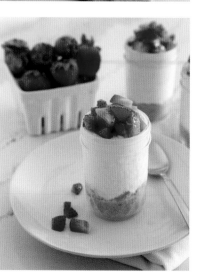
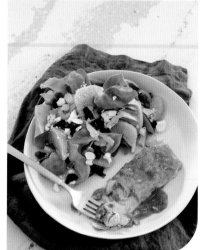

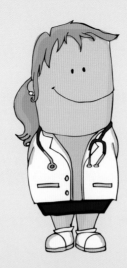

SECTION I

WHAT, WHY, AND HOW OF FODMAP REINTRODUCTION

In section I of this book, I will provide you with background about the low-FODMAP diet and discuss the categories of FODMAPs that you will be challenging, one at a time. I will explain the rationale for reintroducing FODMAPs and review the schedule you should follow. I will reveal many tips for you to succeed! Then I will share simple and delicious low-FODMAP recipes (your "maintenance diet") to keep you stable while you test your tolerances.

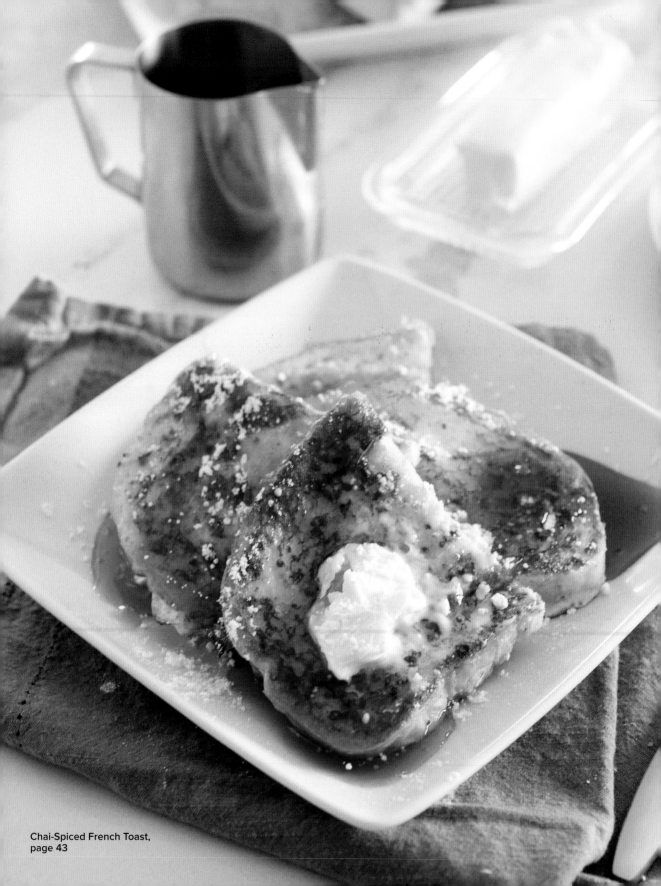

Chai-Spiced French Toast,
page 43

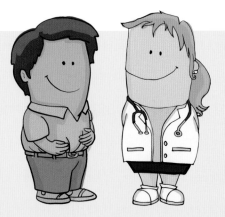

FODMAPS AND REINTRODUCTION
RECLAIM THE FOODS YOU LOVE

FODMAP DIET REVISITED

Let's get started with some background information. The purpose of this book is **not** to start you on the low-FODMAP diet. You have already been following it (I hope!) and have tools that supported the initial stage of your journey. If you don't already own it, I highly recommend my first book, *The Low-FODMAP IBS Solution Plan and Cookbook,* as a great resource.

You are here because you are doing well with the low-FODMAP diet but are wondering what's next for you. Are you going to watch every morsel you put in your mouth forever? Or can you enjoy a taste of onion and garlic from time to time?

Reintroduction (also known as the FODMAP Challenge Phase) provides the answer to those questions. I am going to simplify the process so you can not only *do* it, but also *understand* it. Knowledge is power, friends.

First, however, I will review some basics about the low-FODMAP diet, to make the next steps a bit simpler to follow.

Before we begin, an important note: If the low-FODMAP diet has not been beneficial to you, you may want to spend some time exploring the reasons for that. I do not suggest pursuing reintroduction until your symptoms are well under control. If you've been on the diet for at least 4 weeks and are still experiencing symptoms, take a look at the sidebar titled "Seven Fixes When the Low-FODMAP Diet Fails" and speak to your health care provider for further information.

WHAT IS A FODMAP?

The low-FODMAP diet was first developed by researchers in Australia in the early 2000s. These researchers discovered that certain types of carbohydrates (that span many categories of foods) are more likely to trigger gastrointestinal symptoms such as gas, bloating, diarrhea, and constipation. In short, these carbohydrates, labeled "FODMAPs," are often the triggers for symptoms of IBS.

Their theory? Remove the FODMAPs and you can remove the pain and discomfort associated with IBS.

In the last two decades, numerous studies have confirmed this hypothesis. Research has proven, time and again, that the low-FODMAP diet improves IBS symptoms in more than 80 percent of patients, making it the number one treatment for people suffering from the condition. It helps with IBS-D (diarrhea), IBS-C (constipation), and IBS-M (mixed bowel habits). It is also of benefit in treating gastroparesis, Crohn's, SIBO, and many other digestive disorders. In fact, the American Gastroenterological Association (AGA) recently published a Clinical

Practice Update that states, "The low-FODMAP diet is currently the most evidence-based diet intervention for IBS." It is their recommended first-line dietary therapy in treating the condition.

It's important to remember that the low-FODMAP diet does not *cure* IBS or other conditions. No medical treatment (drug, diet change, or surgery) can do that. But it *can* reduce symptoms and improve quality of life.

You may be familiar with the acronym FODMAP (an acronym is a word where all the first letters stand for something else). **The term does not delineate the different FODMAP categories exactly, but rather serves as an umbrella term.** That is to say, the FODMAP categories are *suggested* by the headings in the acronym, but not clearly called out. You can read the *actual categories* in the table on page 18.

SEVEN FIXES WHEN THE LOW-FODMAP DIET FAILS

The low-FODMAP diet isn't working for you—now what? Before you abandon the low-FODMAP path, try these seven "fixes" to see whether they make a difference.

Fully commit to the program: The elimination phase of the low-FODMAP diet is not something to take lightly. It involves dedication, education, and discipline. If you don't commit 100 percent to following the diet, particularly at first, then you may not see results. You must check the label of *every* food you eat; cook many, if not all, of your meals at your home; and enlist the support of your loved ones.

Make sure you have an accurate low-FODMAP food list: This is central to the whole process. Unfortunately, there are many inaccurate recipes on the internet, out-of-date pamphlets at doctors' offices, and unreliable printed books. Since low-FODMAP food lists are constantly evolving, it is necessary to stay up-to-date with the latest information. I highly recommend purchasing a food app (see "The Apps" page 19) to be your guide to this.

Stick to a correct portion size: This is one of the hardest parts of the diet. What is 30 grams? Is an Australian tablespoon more than a U.S. one? What does one-eighth of an avocado look like when you are eating out? Unfortunately, you must be careful not to overconsume FODMAPs, particularly because everything you eat will "add up" over the day (see "Stacking," page 22). If your symptoms aren't under control, verify your portion sizes (see "Portion Size vs. Serving Size," page 29) to make sure you aren't accidentally eating more FODMAPs than you should.

Read ingredient labels: This is so important. I have assumed numerous times that a food was low FODMAP only to be shocked, after reading the label, to discover it contained onion or garlic (examples: dry-roasted peanuts, crackers, potato chips, spices, and cheese blends). Pay attention;

it is worth that extra minute to glance at the package (see "How to Read Labels," page 26).

Be careful of stacking similar low-FODMAP foods: A food may be low FODMAP, but if you consume your maximum allocation during a meal, then later add another food in the same FODMAP category, you may end up eating too much. To help avoid this common pitfall, I recommend sticking to low-FODMAP recipes such as those in this book, in my first book *The Low-FODMAP IBS Solution Plan and Cookbook,* or at www.rachelpaulsfood.com.

Attend to other IBS triggers that could derail your results: Our bodies do not operate in a vacuum. We move in a world of multiple system interactions. Emotional stress, hormonal variations, and inadequate sleep are just a few triggers that may disrupt our digestion and cause IBS flares. Keep an eye out for these. If possible, reduce other dietary irritants such as sugar, caffeine, carbonation, high-fat foods, and alcohol.

Consider another food intolerance or medical condition: Many people note that while FODMAPs do trigger their IBS, they're not the complete picture. Sometimes people are sensitive to other elements within foods. This could indicate a milk protein allergy, celiac disease, or histamine intolerance. If you suspect one of these conditions might be contributing to your symptoms, discuss with your doctor to determine whether further testing is needed. An anatomic (structural) problem is another possible culprit. These include pelvic organ prolapse and pelvic floor dyssynergia (a condition I specialize in as a urogynecologist). See "Prolapse and Problems with Poop," page 163, for more on this important topic.

FODMAP stands for:

- **F: Fermentable—can be broken down by bacteria in the intestine and made into gas**
- **O: Oligosaccharides—carbohydrates made up of chains of sugars**
- **D: Disaccharides—carbohydrates made of two linked sugars**
- **M: Monosaccharides—carbohydrates made of one sugar**
- **A: and**
- **P: Polyalcohols—sugar alcohols**

The FODMAP categories you will be testing during reintroduction are described indirectly in that acronym. Those of you who use the Monash or FODMAP Friendly apps (see "The Apps," page 19) have seen the six categories of FODMAPs they test and report. You know that FODMAPs span a lot of different "groups" of foods, such as fruits, vegetables, and grains. Some foods also have FODMAPs from *more than one category* (example: watermelon). All of this can make reintroduction very tricky, but if you are reading this book, you have no need to worry. I am going to walk you through it.

The six FODMAP categories you will be testing during reintroduction are listed in the table below.

FODMAP Category	Examples
Oligosaccharides Fructans (oligofructose, inulin, FOS)	wheat, rye, onion, garlic, artichoke
Galacto-oligosaccharides (GOS)	legumes, pulses (chickpeas, beans, lentils), certain nuts
Disaccharides Lactose	milk and milk products
Monosaccharides Fructose (aka excess fructose)	mango, fig, honey, high fructose corn syrup
Polyalcohols (polyols) Sorbitol Mannitol Others: lactitol, xylitol, maltitol, isomalt	stone fruits (peach) cauliflower, celery sugar-free gum and mints

WHY DO FODMAPS TRIGGER IBS?

There are multiple ways this group of foods can trigger GI symptoms, as each category poses its own unique challenges to our bodies' digestion. Fructose, for example, is a sugar that is poorly absorbed in everyone due to a slow transport mechanism in the intestine. Lactose is broken down by the important enzyme *lactase*, which declines with age in about 70 percent of individuals. Polyols are sugar alcohols that diffuse across the gut lining and there is a strict maximum to the amount our systems can handle at any time. Finally, when it comes to fructans and GOS, our bodies simply lack the digestive enzymes to break them down properly.

The bottom line is that FODMAPs trigger gas, bloating, and other symptoms in almost every person who eats them. We've all heard the jokes about beans; well, there is some science behind it. So, why can your friends consume FODMAPs without any symptoms? Why does most of the world incorporate onion and garlic into its cuisine?

The fact is, people with IBS are wired a little differently. Doctors like to use (confusing) words like *visceral hypersensitivity*, *dysmotility*, and *microbiome diversity*. What they mean, essentially, is people with IBS are much more aware of *what goes on* in their intestines. Their intestines move *differently* when digesting food, leading to *more* bloating, *more* discomfort, and *more* symptoms. Finally, the gut of people with IBS may have different *types and proportions of bacteria*, which changes digestive patterns.

Since people with the medical diagnosis of IBS are more sensitive to the gas distention and other symptoms that are triggered by the FODMAP categories, people with IBS react much more profoundly when they consume FODMAPs.

Our bodies are more aware. It's just the way it is. So, let's accept it and embrace the most effective strategies for managing our symptoms. We are in this together!

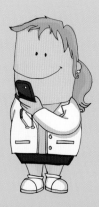

THE APPS

Since you are a seasoned FODMAPPER, you are probably already familiar with the food apps that are available to help guide your food selections. If you are already comfortable with these, then you can read ahead.

For those of you who have been managing exclusively using a book, a printed food list, or the internet, please know that it is *very* worthwhile to purchase a food app for your phone. These apps are much more accurate and up-to-date than anything you'll find online. Not only can you access them anywhere, anytime, but they also include educational elements for the FODMAP journey and beyond.

The two apps that I suggest purchasing are the Monash University app and the FODMAP Friendly app. You can learn more at www. monashfodmap.com/ibs-central/i-have-ibs/get-the-app and www.fodmapfriendly.com/app.

Both apps are reliable resources, but we will be using the Monash app more frequently in this book. That is because they have a larger food list in their database, and they have been reporting in this format longer.

Occasionally, foods will have slightly different FODMAP values between Monash and FODMAP Friendly. There are many reasons for this. For one, foods are variable in their seasonality, ripeness, and growth location. Both companies test foods at a given time, using a given number of foods for a sampling. They cannot possibly test EVERY apple from EVERY geographical origin. Naturally, this results in variation. Please do not let these differences cause you anxiety. You can always use the more stringent result to guide your menu choices and test your tolerance to that particular food.

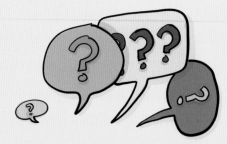

FODMAP FAQS

Here are my answers to common queries about the low-FODMAP diet, to help you succeed when reintroducing foods.

Q: I don't understand how soy is sometimes low FODMAP and sometimes high FODMAP. Can you explain that?
A: This *is* a confusing product category! The reason behind the differences among FODMAP levels in soy products relates to when and how the soy is processed. Let's take a closer look:

- Mature whole soybeans contain the fiber from the soy, which is high in GOS and fructans. Therefore, foods made with mature whole soybeans are high in FODMAPs.

  + Examples: soy milk made with whole soybeans, and soy flour

- Immature whole soybeans are picked before they have finished ripening, so their FODMAP content is lower than mature soybeans.

  + Example: edamame

- Soy protein is available *without* the FODMAP-containing fiber and may be lower in FODMAPs.

  + Example: soy milk made with soy protein

- Soaking soy for a long time will leach the FODMAPs from the final product, so it will cause fewer digestive issues.

  + Examples: tempeh, extra-firm tofu

- Soy processing that does not involve this soaking process is not low FODMAP.

  + Examples: soft and silken tofu

- Fermenting soybeans reduces the FODMAP content.

  + Example: soy sauce

Q: Why are ripe bananas and unripe bananas different in FODMAP content?
A: Bananas, like soy, have alterations in FODMAP content depending on their maturity. A green, unripe banana is made up of about 80 percent starches. As it ripens, however, the starches convert to sugars, which contain the offending FODMAPs (in this case, fructans). Thus, if the banana is very ripe, you cannot consume more than one-third of a medium-size fruit (35 g).

Q: Why can I have onion-infused oil, but not use onion in my chicken soup, if I don't eat the onion itself?
A: Great question. It has to do with the fact that FODMAPs are soluble (dissolve) in water, but not in oil. Even if you remove the pieces of onion from your soup, the onion's FODMAPs have already leached out into the water-based liquid of the soup broth. However, if you stick to adding a little bit of onion-infused oil after the soup is cooked, then you will have the onion flavor, but not the stomachache.

Q: How are butter and Cheddar cheese allowed in low-FODMAP recipes, yet I can't have milk and ice cream?

A: Milk and milk products' FODMAP content is based on the amount of lactose in the food. So dairy products that contain less lactose will contain fewer FODMAPs. Cheese, butter, and cream have less lactose (since they are lower in carbohydrate content) and thus can be consumed based on their allocated serving size. Milk and ice cream have higher amounts of lactose and should be avoided until you reach that stage of reintroduction.

Q: Can you explain sourdough bread? Is it low FODMAP or not?

A: Sourdough bread is made using a unique process that involves bacterial fermentation. The fermentation process, if of suitable duration (overnight), will result in conversion of the fructans in the wheat to a more digestible form. Current data suggests this is limited to white, wheat, or spelt flour sourdough breads. Be aware that those breads still contain gluten, so they should be avoided in cases of celiac disease or gluten sensitivity.

Q: What is the story behind corn? Why can I have large amounts of some corn products, but not others?

A: Corn varies in FODMAP content, depending on the type of corn you consume. Field corn (also known as dent corn) is typically used for corn flour and cornmeal and is lower in FODMAPs than sweet corn on the cob. Popcorn is another variety of corn that is typically low FODMAP in standard servings. Finally, canning corn can cause FODMAPs to leach away with the liquid in the canning juice, and thus a rinsed and drained canned product is often selected for my recipes.

REINTRODUCTION: AN OVERVIEW

Reintroduction is the second phase of the low-FODMAP journey. The purpose of this phase is to identify the types and amounts of FODMAPs that you can tolerate, so you can add them back to your everyday diet. It is also sometimes also referred to as the *FODMAP Challenge Phase*.

This process, if done correctly, will take time. Each FODMAP category is introduced at a low level and gradually increased over a three-day period. The three-day period may occur over three consecutive days, followed by three "break" or "washout" days, or on alternating days, with a "break" or "washout" day in between. That plan will vary based on the FODMAP category you are testing.

While you are doing these challenges, it is important to stay on a strict, low-FODMAP "maintenance" diet—like the one you followed during the elimination phase—for all other meals. This is your baseline. Keeping to this diet through the reintroduction process means you won't be confused about what triggers your symptoms. As you may recall, symptoms don't always happen immediately after consuming a FODMAP trigger; rather, they can happen toward the end of the day as the food moves through your digestive symptom (see "Stacking," at right).

Eventually, if you do well with all the individual food challenges, you will start testing "combination" foods. Those are foods that contain more than one FODMAP category. Moving toward those combination foods will enable you to begin integration and personalization of the FODMAP diet, or phase 3.

If it sounds like a big commitment, well, it is. But don't be intimidated. Remember, you have complete oversight and control of the process. If you only want to test a few foods, such as the ones you are more likely to eat at restaurants, then do that. If you want to take breaks between challenges, go for it! You set the pace, and you decide. I am here to make the journey as easy as possible.

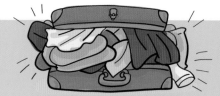

STACKING

Over the course of the day, everything we eat eventually makes it to our intestines. The small and large intestines together are approximately 15 feet (4.6 m) long, so this trip can take a while. As a result, the foods you eat accumulate, depending on the speed of your digestion and the type of food they are. This is called *stacking*.

Food stacking is one of the reasons that it can be tricky to know which foods are triggering your IBS. It isn't usually the food that you *just ate* causing your gas or bloating, but the breakfast you ate that morning, plus the snack you ate a few hours ago, that is causing your problems. This is one of the reasons why journaling your symptoms over the course of a day or longer is so helpful. (See page 33 for more information about the timing of GI symptoms relative to meals.)

I like to use this analogy to describe stacking: Imagine your intestines are a suitcase that you are packing with clothes (food). At first, the suitcase is comfortable and light. But as you continue to pack it with clothes, it becomes more and more distended. Suddenly it's bursting apart at the seams. That is what happens in your gut over the course of the day if you eat foods that are not easily digested.

WHY REINTRODUCTION MATTERS

I hear you asking, why should I even bother?

It sounds like a lot of time and effort, and you are feeling so good right now, you don't want that to change.

I totally understand both sentiments. It took me a long time to work up the courage to reintroduce. But there are many benefits.

First and foremost, reintroduction will improve your personal freedom. We're all familiar with the obstacles that the low-FODMAP diet creates in daily life. There are fewer options when eating out, the potential to feel restricted in social situations, and extra difficulties while traveling. Through reintroduction you might learn that you can tolerate lactose, modest amounts of bread, small amounts of onion and garlic, and other FODMAPs, thereby significantly expanding your options in these situations.

Another benefit is simply the pleasure you take in your food. We all gave up some of our favorite foods when we started the low-FODMAP diet. This is a great opportunity to discover whether you can go back to eating them! Missing your mango salsa or avocado toast? You may learn that you can add those culinary delights back into your regular routine (see pages 113 and 121 for recipes).

Reintroducing foods is also a step toward optimal gut health. Food diversity is necessary for digestive wellness. Adding back some of the higher FODMAP foods will improve your gut's "microbiome" (see "The Intestinal Microbiome," below), which can have a positive impact on your mood and immune system. Furthermore, eating a wide variety of foods offers the best overall nutritional balance, ensuring you consume the correct vitamins, minerals, and amino acids your body needs.

Finally, reintroduction offers guidance for planning your future. Once you have your personal tolerances clarified, you will be well on your way to beginning your long-term "Modified" or "Personalized" low-FODMAP eating plan. This will be your future reality. A strict low-FODMAP diet should not be forever.

THE INTESTINAL MICROBIOME

The intestinal microbiome describes the unique array of organisms that live in our digestive tracts, including bacteria, fungi, and yeasts. These organisms "colonize" our organs, but don't cause us harm (as opposed to the types of bacteria that cause infections, or for which we take antibiotics). Not only do the bacteria in the microbiome help digest food, but they also release hormones and chemicals that balance our mood and boost our immunity.

Each person's intestines have a special and unique microbiome, although there are similarities within populations and cultures. Your microbiome depends on your diet to a large degree, and other factors in your health.

We know that having a diverse microbiome is beneficial. What we also know is that *probiotic* bacteria are good for us, which is why you've probably heard about taking probiotics to help your health (see page 161). Well, the probiotic bacteria in our intestines like to consume *prebiotic* fiber. Prebiotic fiber often comes from high-FODMAP foods such as onion, garlic, and asparagus.

In other words, eating foods that are prebiotic helps the probiotic bacteria in our gut flourish and thereby improves our microbiome diversity. Foods that contain higher levels of FODMAPs are a key part of that process. Consequently, attempting to reintroduce those foods is strongly recommended by doctors and health care providers.

STRATEGIES FOR SUCCESS

When is the best time to begin reintroduction? Only you know the answer to that. If you decide to complete all the challenges consecutively, with no interruptions, then it should take around three months. However, I suggest (for practical reasons) planning some breaks in that schedule.

Reintroduction requires you to be strict about your low-FODMAP adherence on the days surrounding and including your testing day. That is the only way to ensure that you aren't having a symptom flare related to another FODMAP category. This can create some limitations in your personal and professional life. I don't endorse completing the challenges during a vacation, work conference, or family event. It could lead to frustration and early burnout.

Speaking of food limitations, I suggest that you be careful about other gut triggers that are not FODMAPs. If you are sensitive to fat, sugar, caffeine, alcohol, or carbonation, then keep away from those during testing days. I also recommend avoiding challenges on days at higher risk for a flare. For example, my hormonal cycle is a big contributor to my IBS tolerance (see "Menstruation, Menopause, and IBS," page 25). Finally, for the best results, try to limit stress and aim for adequate sleep, always good advice when trying to avoid an IBS flare-up.

Some other tips for reintroduction:

- **Adhere to my recommended challenge foods:** The foods you use to challenge each FODMAP category are very specific and should not be altered. Unless you are highly familiar with the nutritional profile of your proposed alternative, you could accidentally end up testing more than one FODMAP category at a time (example: apples contain both fructose and sorbitol). This misinformation could derail your results if you reacted to the food, because you won't know which component triggered you.

- **Be mindful of your symptoms:** Because IBS varies from person to person, it is important to acknowledge what a flare-up is for you. Perhaps it's diarrhea, constipation, or bloating. Record symptoms as they occur to carefully track your progress. In fact, I recommend journaling throughout the entire reintroduction process. This may mean writing in a notebook or computer. Or perhaps you prefer taking notes on your phone because it's easily accessible. Whatever works! Just keep track of what your reactions are and when they happen. This will help guide your transition to the next challenge. See figures 1 and 2, pages 31 and 32, for sample journal entries.

- **Break days are necessary:** Don't skip break/washout days! These are included for a reason, to cleanse and balance your system. Take advantage of the time between challenges to pay attention to your body and prepare for the next food category. For certain categories, break days are strategically placed between challenge days, to give your gut longer to react. Planned breaks can also sleuth out any flares unrelated to your FODMAP adjustments, thereby indicating a need to retest a food later when you are feeling your best.

- **Stop challenges if needed:** If you start to experience symptoms at any time during a challenge, STOP that challenge immediately. Remember, there is no deadline. The most important thing is to be certain of your reactions, and the best way to do that is to *pause and reset*. The worst thing you could do is push forward, cause a larger flare, and negatively impact your desire to continue.

- **Set up a support network:** Get others invested in your plan. Talk to your friends, family, and coworkers. If you have a dietitian, then ask for their support and additional guidance. This will be a lengthy process, and you don't have to do it alone.

- **Stick to a low-FODMAP maintenance diet:** Don't stray from your low-FODMAP diet now! I know we all have "cheat" moments/days/weekends, but try to minimize them while performing the challenges. You want your body functioning at its best so you can correctly interpret its reactions. To help, I have provided a suggested meal plan and many new low-FODMAP recipes that you can try. Be sure to always *read labels* (see "How to Read Labels," page 26) and be wary of any other food triggers.

- **Pace yourself:** Take this process at your own pace. You may want to challenge two FODMAP categories, then take a month off and start again. Whatever feels right. Just put this book on the shelf and pick it up when you're ready. You are not committing to any specific schedule other than your own.

- **Be patient with the process:** As much as you may want to reintroduce high-FODMAP foods that you have tolerated in prior challenges as you move to the next phase of your journey, I don't recommend it. You should continue to limit the number of FODMAPs in your testing days to achieve the best results. Later in this journey we will test "combination" foods, and that will let you know whether you are okay with two or more FODMAPs in one sitting. Sound good? Let's begin!

MENSTRUATION, MENOPAUSE, AND IBS

If you are reading this as a person who menstruates or has menstruated, then you may have noticed that your hormonal cycle impacts the severity of your IBS. Symptoms may worsen just before or during your period, a process known as *menstrual magnification*. If you are peri- or postmenopausal, fluctuating levels of hormones could be wreaking havoc on your gut harmony.

I have two blogs on my website, www.rachelpaulsfood.com, that discuss these issues in more detail: "Does Menopause Worsen Irritable Bowel Syndrome (IBS)? Dr. Rachel's Top 10 Tips to Help Symptoms" and "IBS and PMS, The Daunting Duo; Dr. Rachel Pauls's Top 7 Tips for Dealing with Symptoms."

If you think this is happening to you, know that you are not alone. Some great ways to manage elevated symptoms during these times include getting enough sleep, limiting stress, exercising, doing meditation, and practicing yoga. Abdominal wall massage and heating packs are also very handy during your periods to help control your pain (see "Tummy-Taming Techniques," page 119).

When it comes to reintroduction, I suggest pausing the process while your hormonal environment is unstable. It may be difficult to accurately record the relationship between symptoms and trigger foods during this time, not to mention the extra toll it takes on your body. This might mean performing FODMAP challenges only in the three weeks after your period or waiting until menopausal symptoms subside. Either way, this is YOUR journey, and it is not a race. The goal is for you to obtain the most accurate information possible. That is what makes the experience a success.

HOW TO READ LABELS

Becoming an expert at identifying high-FODMAP triggers will help keep your symptoms under control. Understanding how to read food labels is a key part of the process.

For starters, ingredients in a food label are listed in order of weight. So, the item listed first has the highest weight in the product, and the last item may only be a tiny fraction of the product. That can be helpful, for example, for a food that lists onion powder as the last ingredient. The actual amount of onion powder could be so small that you can tolerate it, even though it wouldn't seem to qualify as low FODMAP.

Next, you may come across certain items that do not appear on any approved low-FODMAP lists. If you haven't heard of it, and can't find out what it is, then don't eat it!

Below are some low-FODMAP and high-FODMAP additives to be aware of. Remember, always check your food app (see "The Apps," page 19) for the most up-to-date information.

LOW-FODMAP ADDITIVES (THESE ARE OKAY TO CONSUME):

- Almond extract
- Apple cider vinegar
- Asafoetida spice
- Aspartame
- Baking powder
- Baking soda
- Balsamic vinegar
- Brown sugar
- Buckwheat
- Cane juice
- Cane juice crystals
- Cane sugar
- Carrageenan
- Cellulose
- Citric acid
- Cocoa
- Confectioners' (icing) sugar
- Corn syrup (not high-fructose variety)
- Cornstarch
- Glucose
- Guar gum
- Locust bean gum
- Malt extract
- Maltose
- Maple syrup
- Miso paste
- Modified food starch
- Pectin
- Potato starch
- Resistant starch
- Rice flour
- Rice protein
- Rice wine vinegar
- Saccharin
- Soy lecithin
- Soy sauce
- Soybean oil
- Stevia
- Sucralose
- Sucrose
- Sugar
- Tapioca flour
- Tapioca starch
- Vanilla extract
- Wasabi
- Wheat dextrin
- Wheat starch
- Xanthan gum

HIGH-FODMAP ADDITIVES (THESE YOU SHOULD AVOID):

- Agave syrup
- Barley
- Chickpea flour
- Chicory root fiber
- Coconut treacle
- Crystalline fructose
- Dehydrated vegetables
- Dried fruits
- Dry milk solids
- Fructans
- Fructo-oligosaccharides (FOS)
- Fructose and fructose solids
- Fructose-glucose syrup
- Fruit juice concentrate
- Garlic powder
- Gluco-oligosaccharides (GOS)
- Glucose-fructose syrup
- Glycerin/glycerol
- Golden syrup
- High-fructose corn syrup
- Honey
- Hydrogenated starch hydrolysates
- Inulin
- Isoglucose
- Isomalt
- Kamut
- Lactitol
- Lactulose
- Maltitol
- Mannitol
- Milk solids
- Molasses
- Onion extract
- Onion powder
- Polydextrose
- Rye
- Sorbitol
- Soy nuts
- Soybeans, whole
- Xylitol
- Yacon syrup

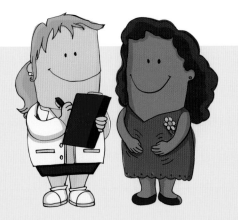

REINTRODUCTION:
THE DETAILS

GETTING STARTED

The reintroduction phase of the low-FODMAP diet is much more flexible than the elimination phase. Isn't that a refreshing change? You can follow your instincts, set personal goals, and structure the challenges according to your own preferences.

For many of the FODMAP categories, you will select which food you want to use as your test. To test fructose, for example, you could choose honey, mango, or asparagus.

The schedule for the challenges is also modifiable by you. However, I provide a sequence for testing that I recommend in which reintroduction is broken into three stages. My sequence moves through the FODMAP categories in an order that you are most likely to tolerate (meaning fewer flares). Following this pattern has been associated with higher success and will hopefully encourage you to keep going!

What time of day should you test? It's up to you! But I suggest you pick a preferred time of day for each challenge and stick to that time for all three test days (though ideally for the entire reintroduction process). I also endorse completing the full challenge amount in one sitting, rather than spreading it out over the day. Consuming the challenge food in conjunction with a meal, combined with other foods, is ideal because it replicates your future behavior. My personal preference is to test earlier, for breakfast or lunch, but that is not mandatory.

You are going to start the first day with a moderate dose of the food, then increase to a high dose on the second test day, and end with a very high dose on the last challenge day (see "Portion Size vs. Serving Size," page 29).

For many of the challenges in stage 1, feel free to complete the three test days all in a row. However, when testing the more complex fructans and GOS in stage 2, I suggest spacing these with a day in between. That is because those FODMAPs may be slower to move through your digestive tract. If you have IBS-constipation, alternating test days with break days may be your preferred schedule throughout the process.

For each challenge, I will provide you with one or more delicious recipes involving a challenge food. Of course, you may use a different recipe incorporating that food or enjoy the food on its own.

Some good news for those of you who have the Monash app (see "The Apps," page 19). The Monash app has a place where you can see options for reintroduction foods and their recommended serving sizes (in grams). To find this information, click the "Diary," then the "+" symbol in the upper right. Next, click the pictorial of the apple with a circling arrow around it, select your subgroup, and the options should populate.

I don't recommend mixing and matching food choices in the three test days (for example, eating honey for the fructose test during days 1 and 2 and then using mango for the last test). It may not escalate the amount appropriately. You could also be reacting to something other than the FODMAP in the new food. I encourage you to stick to the same test food for all three challenge days, for the clearest results.

If you prefer your food choice cooked, then that is fine. Depending on the food, the recommended weight may change with cooking. As a rule, if the food can be consumed raw (like celery), then the weight for the challenge will be the raw weight. You should weigh the amount *before* cooking. However, for foods that are usually eaten cooked (like pasta), the challenge weight will be the cooked weight. That is typically how Monash reports their FODMAP levels, and that will be our standard in guiding these measurements. If you are ever unsure, then you can't go wrong using the raw weight, as the cooked weight will typically be lower (which could result in you eating *too much* of that food).

The result you document from each FODMAP test is intended to reflect your sensitivity to that entire FODMAP category. In other words, if you document during the fructose challenge that you tolerate honey, then you should be able to enjoy any food that contains a similar amount of fructose (such as a tomato). However, remember that factors *other than FODMAPs* trigger GI symptoms. It is possible that you could react negatively to a tomato if you are sensitive to high-acid foods. Be aware of your personal medical circumstances prior to widely increasing your consumption.

It may seem like a lot to remember. Don't worry! As long as you "follow your gut," you will achieve success!

PORTION SIZE VS. SERVING SIZE

Portion size is an important consideration in beginning and maintaining control on the low-FODMAP diet. Most of you are already aware that almost *any* food can be tolerated, provided a *small enough* portion is eaten. The exact amount of that portion differs from person to person and is something you will be establishing when you reintroduce.

The portion sizes I am using in this book are those recommended by the Monash app as low FODMAP, or suitable escalations for reintroduction. That does not mean that you will or will not have IBS symptoms with that food portion. However, it provides a feasible structure for our testing, and a starting point.

A portion size may be much smaller than a "typical" serving of that food. Or it may be much more than you would usually consume. For example, the maximum testing portion size for cashews I will outline is 45 g, or about 1.5 ounces. That is a 250-calorie serving of cashews—an amount that you may regularly wish to eat, or way more than you would ever choose. If it is not a desirable portion for you to consume, or you don't tolerate nuts for another reason, then select a different option for that challenge. There will be other choices for you!

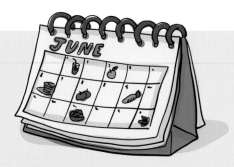

YOUR REINTRODUCTION TOOLKIT

Journal

This can be a paper and pen journal, an Excel file, or a note-taking app on your phone. Use whichever system is most convenient for you, but don't skip this step! It is critical that you thoroughly document each challenge day so you have a record of how your body responds. See figure 1 on page 31 and figure 2 on page 32 for a sample journal entry to get you started.

Monash and FODMAP Friendly apps

I suggest purchasing both of the above apps. If you have to pick only one, then I recommend Monash, simply because it has a larger number of foods in its database. These are an invaluable resource to guide you on the low-FODMAP diet (see "The Apps," page 19).

Food scale

A necessity in every kitchen. My FODMAP category challenges list the portion sizes by weight in *grams* because this is the *most accurate method* to ensure you're consuming the correct amount of FODMAPs. Simply stating "one-half" of a celery stalk or "¼ cup" of chickpeas is not precise enough. The Monash University and FODMAP Friendly apps are both based in Australia, so they usually delineate portion sizes in grams as well.

REINTRODUCTION, STAGE I

For the first stage of reintroduction, you will be testing fructose, lactose, and the polyols sorbitol and mannitol. Before you begin, I recommend you complete three days of *maintenance* or *baseline* low-FODMAP eating to get your system ready for testing. These FODMAP categories will follow a schedule of three consecutive challenge days followed by three *break* or *washout* days.

Remember, it is important to carefully follow your low-FODMAP diet during your break days and ensure that you keep track of your symptoms with a journal. This will allow you to note whether the new food is responsible for any changes in your symptoms.

Here is my suggested sequence for reintroduction, stage 1 testing, followed by a sample journal entry documenting one of these challenges:

- **Low-FODMAP maintenance diet (3 days)**
- **Fructose testing (3 days)**
- **Break (at least 3 days)**
- **Lactose testing (3 days)**
- **Break (at least 3 days)**
- **Polyols: sorbitol testing (3 days)**
- **Break (at least 3 days)**
- **Polyols: mannitol testing (3 days)**
- **Break (at least 3 days)**

FIGURE 1. SAMPLE JOURNAL ENTRY FOR STAGE I CHALLENGES

	Sorbitol Challenge	Symptoms	Other Notes
CHALLENGE DAY 1	Avocado, 40 g (sliced on sandwich with smoked turkey)	None	Good day!
CHALLENGE DAY 2	Avocado, 80 g (Perfect Avocado Toast, page 121)	None	Stayed up late to finish work presentation
CHALLENGE DAY 3	Avocado, 120 g (added extra to Quinoa Power Bowl with Southwest Dressing, page 53)	None	Presentation to clients, went well
BREAK DAY 4	Low-FODMAP diet only	Feeling good	Saturday, busy day with kids
BREAK DAY 5	Low-FODMAP diet only	Feeling good	Sunday, went for hike
BREAK DAY 6	Low-FODMAP diet only	Feeling good	Normal workday

FINDINGS: Tolerated 120 g avocado for sorbitol challenge; some stressors but didn't trigger flare

REINTRODUCTION, STAGE 2

In stage 2 of reintroduction, you will be testing fructans and GOS. These subtypes tend to be harder to digest for most people. They move more slowly through our systems, thus IBS flares may not show up as quickly. For that reason, I recommend having a break day *between* test days, rather than testing over three consecutive days.

You will continue to record any symptom changes in your journal. If you have discomfort, then stop the challenge with that amount and move on to the break period.

Finally, if you never intend to eat a test food, you can skip that challenge. For example, if you are gluten-intolerant, then you would omit the wheat challenge altogether.

At right is my suggested sequence (test days will alternate with break days), followed by a sample journal entry for one of the challenges.

- Low-FODMAP maintenance diet (3 days)
- Fructans, vegetables, and fruits testing (6 days with breaks)
- Fructans, wheat testing (6 days with breaks)
- Fructans, onion testing (6 days with breaks)
- Fructans, garlic testing (6 days with breaks)
- GOS testing (6 days with breaks)

FIGURE 2. SAMPLE JOURNAL ENTRY FOR STAGE 2 CHALLENGES

	GOS Challenge	Symptoms	Other Notes
CHALLENGE DAY 1	Chickpeas, 84 g (added to mixed greens salad)	None	Saturday, getting over a cold
BREAK DAY 1	Low-FODMAP diet only	None	Sunday, rested; still congested
CHALLENGE DAY 2	Chickpeas, 112 g (Chickpea and Potato Soup, page 149)	None	Cold much better
BREAK DAY 2	Low-FODMAP diet only	None	Doing well
CHALLENGE DAY 3	Chickpeas, 168 g (mashed with lemon juice, infused oil, and sea salt; spread on toast)	Bloating at end of day	Early meeting
BREAK DAY 3	Low-FODMAP diet only	Worse bloating, diarrhea	Normal workday

FINDINGS: Tolerated 112 g chickpeas for GOS challenge; no other stressors

REINTRODUCTION, STAGE 3: FODMAP COMBINATION FOODS

During this stage, you will be consuming foods that include more than one FODMAP subtype. We refer to these as "combination foods." This may sound trickier, but don't worry. I will provide selections for these challenges and suitable recipes.

For this more complex stage, I suggest continuing the pattern of a break day between challenge days. However, you can opt to do all three test days in a row if you prefer.

At right is my recommended sequence of testing for this stage.

- **Low-FODMAP** maintenance diet (3 days)
- **Sorbitol and fructose testing (6 days with breaks)**
- **GOS** and fructans testing (6 days with breaks)
- **Fructans and fructose testing (6 days with breaks)**
- **Sorbitol and fructans testing (6 days with breaks)**

HOW LONG DOES IT TAKE FOR GI SYMPTOMS TO APPEAR AFTER EATING?

Many of us know that food is often the trigger for our IBS symptoms. What we are not good at is understanding *which food* caused them. That is because the time between eating the food and experiencing symptoms can vary greatly. Often, it is not immediate, because food moves from our stomach to the small intestine first, then to the large intestine, where the majority of symptoms occur.

If a response to a food occurs very quickly, such as within 5 to 15 minutes of consumption, it's usually related to an allergic reaction. This is different from a digestive, or FODMAP-triggered, problem. If you eat a peanut and then immediately start having nausea and diarrhea, you are probably allergic to peanuts.

If a response occurs within 15 and 90 minutes after eating, it is usually related to the food reaching the small intestine (the first stop following the stomach). This occurs from time to time in everyone, but is more common in people with an *accelerated* gastrocolic reflex (for more on this, see "Optimize Your Eating Style," page 165). Symptoms include diarrhea and the feeling

that food "runs right through you," if you have IBS-D. Symptoms could also including gurgling, bloating, distention, and gas pain, if you suffer from IBS-C.

In most cases, however, a response to a food occurs when it hits the large intestine. This takes between 2 and 8 hours, a much longer amount of time. Gas, bloating, and loose stools are caused by the poorly absorbed food bolus being broken down by the abundance of bacteria in that organ. Resulting symptoms could be more profound if you have IBS.

YOUR MAINTENANCE DIET DURING REINTRODUCTION

During reintroduction, it's important to remember that although you're entering a new phase of your low-FODMAP journey, your regular, daily diet will not change. Other than the challenge foods, you will continue to follow your low-FODMAP elimination phase diet for several weeks until you complete all your desired categories of testing. I like to call this your "maintenance" or "baseline" diet.

Your maintenance diet can be made up of the food lists, trusted recipes, and preferred menus that you used throughout the elimination phase. If these options kept you stable for the last few weeks, they will continue to keep you stable now. However, if you're ready to try something different, the following chapter has you covered with some great new recipes to add options to your low-FODMAP diet.

I create all my low-FODMAP recipes to be easy, tasty, and good for you. Many of the entrées use only one pot, skillet, or sheet pan to make cleanup a breeze. Your family and friends will never know they are eating gluten-free and low-FODMAP meals.

For even more recipes and snack ideas, my website at www.rachelpaulsfood.com has more than 500 free low-FODMAP recipes and a line of convenient lab-certified low-FODMAP food products such as energy bars (Happy Bars), soup bases (Happy Soup), spice blends (Happy Spices), and baking mixes (Happy Baking).

It is very likely that you will run into conflicts with your personal life, travel plans, and social/work events at some point during the reintroduction phase. There is nothing wrong with pausing your schedule at those times. I suggest taking three to seven days after the event to allow your symptoms to level out before restarting testing.

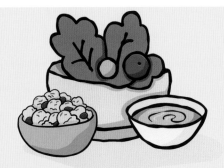

MAINTENANCE DIET

SIMPLE AND DELICIOUS LOW-FODMAP RECIPES

RECIPE ICONS

 Vegan

 Vegetarian

 Gluten Free

 Dairy Free

 Under 5 Ingredients

Yield: 16 biscuits   **Prep time: 10 minutes**   **Bake time: 12 to 15 minutes**

MINI PUMPKIN BISCUITS WITH CREAM CHEESE FROSTING

These scrumptious, flaky mini biscuits can be served for breakfast, as a snack, or for dessert. I adore the flavor of pumpkin spice in baked goods. Try these with my cream cheese frosting and you will have a smile on your face all morning.

FOR THE BISCUITS:

2 cups (240 g) all-purpose gluten-free pancake or biscuit mix, such as Gluten-Free Bisquick*

2 tablespoons (12 g) granulated sugar

¼ teaspoon salt

1 large egg

⅓ cup (85 g) canned pure pumpkin

2 tablespoons (30 ml) low-FODMAP milk, such as lactose-free or almond milk

½ teaspoon vanilla extract

1½ teaspoons pumpkin pie spice

5 tablespoons (75 g) unsalted butter, melted

FOR THE CREAM CHEESE FROSTING:

¼ cup (60 g) lactose-free cream cheese

¼ cup (60 g) unsalted butter, softened

1½ cups (180 g) confectioners' sugar

¼ teaspoon vanilla extract

1 to 2 tablespoons (15 to 30 ml) low-FODMAP milk, such as lactose-free or almond milk

To make the biscuits: Preheat the oven to 400°F (200°C, or gas mark 6), and place a rack in the center of the oven. Line an 11 x 16-inch (27 x 40 cm) baking sheet with a silicone mat or parchment paper, or spray with nonstick spray.

In a large mixing bowl, combine the pancake/biscuit mix, granulated sugar, and salt. In a separate bowl, whisk the egg and pumpkin together, then add the milk, vanilla, and pumpkin pie spice and whisk until combined. Add the pumpkin mixture to the dry ingredients and stir to combine. Finally, add the melted butter and mix until incorporated (you may wish to use your hands at this point to help it stay together).

Use a small ice cream scoop to drop 16 biscuits onto the cookie sheet, about 1 inch (2.5 cm) apart. If the dough is overly crumbly, you may smooth out the tops of the biscuits with your hands, flattening them slightly. Bake for 12 to 15 minutes until the biscuits are lightly golden and the tops are set. Remove from the oven and cool on the sheet for 5 minutes, then transfer to a cooling rack.

To make the frosting: While the biscuits are baking, use an electric mixer to beat the cream cheese with the butter. Slowly add the confectioners' sugar, beating well after each addition. Add the vanilla and mix. Add the milk, 1 teaspoon at a time, beating well, until the frosting reaches your desired consistency. For a thinner frosting, use more milk. If serving the biscuits warm, drizzle with the frosting and enjoy immediately. For later serving, allow the biscuits to cool to room temperature before frosting. Store leftover frosting in the refrigerator for 5 days or freeze for 1 month.

*Check the label to make sure this is made up of only low-FODMAP ingredients.

VARIATION: For a dairy-free frosting, use my vanilla glaze recipe on page 48 instead of the cream cheese frosting here.

NUTRITION PER SERVING: Serving Size: 51 g, Calories: 180, Total Fat: 9 g, Saturated Fat: 5 g, Carbohydrates: 25 g, Sugar: 13 g, Sodium: 180 mg, Fiber: 1 g, Protein: 1 g

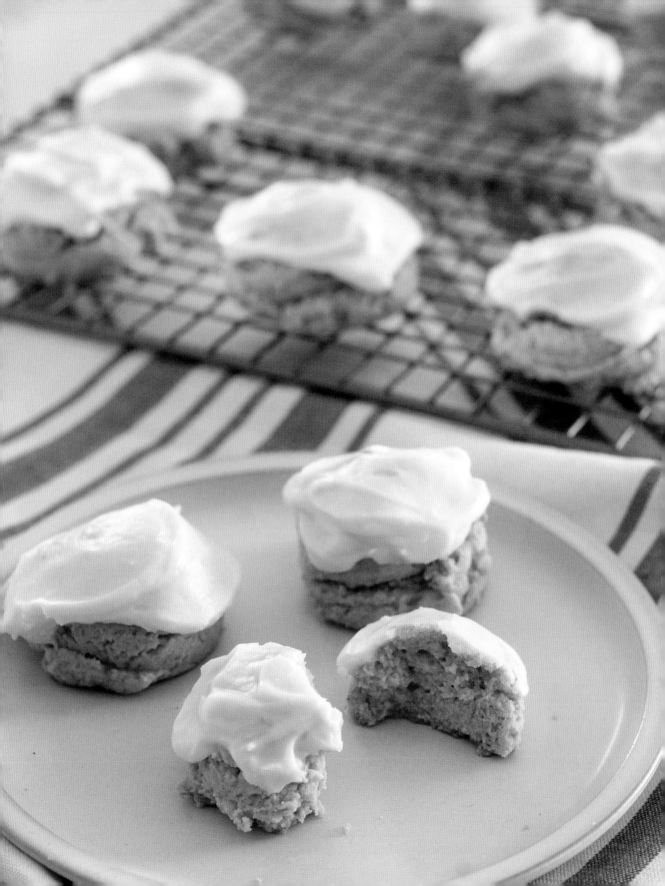

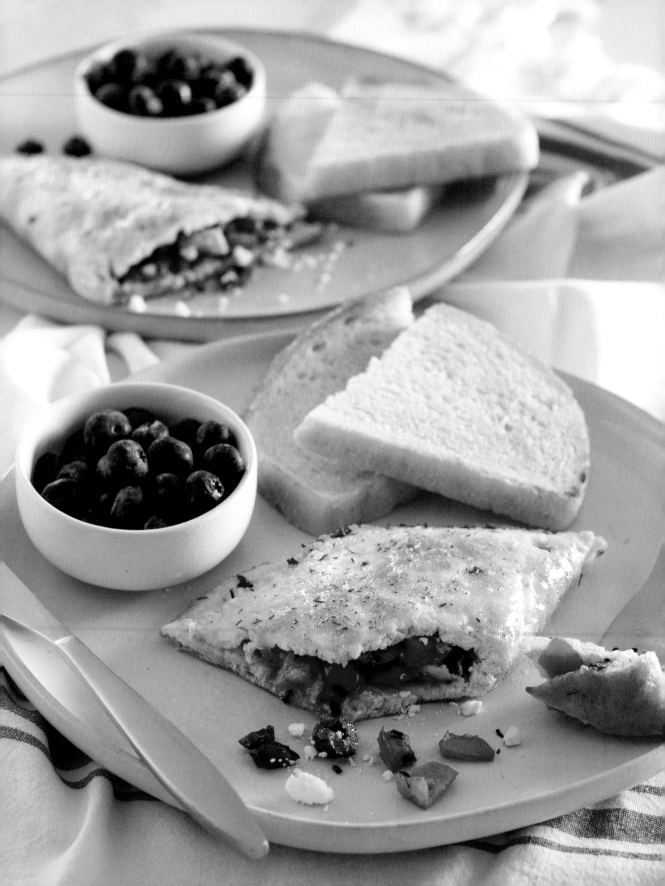

ZESTY GREEK OMELET

My first date with my husband was at a Greek restaurant; we both love Mediterranean cuisine. This omelet is an ideal showcase for the mouthwatering combination of sharp feta, salty olives, and ripe tomatoes. Serve it with a low-FODMAP, gluten-free bagel or fried potatoes.

In a medium bowl, whisk the eggs until well combined. Place a large cast-iron or nonstick saucepan over medium heat and add the oil. When the oil is shimmering, turn the heat down to low and add the olives and chives. Stir until these are warmed through, 2 to 3 minutes, and then remove to a covered dish. Add the eggs to the pan and adjust the heat to medium-low. Once the eggs are slightly cooked on the edges, sprinkle the feta cheese over the omelet, turn the heat to low, and cover the skillet for 3 to 4 minutes. When the cheese and eggs are starting to cook through, sprinkle in the olive mixture, then add the tomatoes on top, and fold the omelet in half. Cook for 1 to 2 minutes more, then plate and sprinkle with the oregano, salt, and pepper to taste. Serve with low-FODMAP, gluten-free toast or bagel and fruit.

VARIATION: If you don't have kalamata olives, you can substitute canned black olives. The flavor will be different, but still delicious.

TIP: Feta cheese is quite salty, so be sure to taste your omelet prior to adding extra salt. You may not need any.

4 large eggs, at room temperature

2 tablespoons (30 ml) canola oil, or your preferred oil for frying

¼ cup (45 g) chopped kalamata olives

2 tablespoons (6 g) chopped chives or green scallion tips

½ cup (60 g) crumbled feta cheese

½ cup (100 g) chopped tomatoes

½ teaspoon dried oregano

Salt and pepper to taste

NUTRITION PER SERVING: Serving Size: 220 g, Calories: 420, Total Fat: 36 g, Saturated Fat: 9 g, Carbohydrates: 6 g, Sugar: 3 g, Sodium: 780 mg, Fiber: 1 g, Protein: 17 g

CARROT CAKE BREAKFAST COOKIES

A cross between a healthy snack and a sweet treat, my carrot cake breakfast cookies are packed with oats, seeds, fresh carrots, and nuts. You can make them completely unsweetened, or amp up the maple syrup for more of a dessert experience. I often bring these to events and they disappear!

1½ cups (120 g) traditional (old-fashioned) rolled oats

⅔ cup (80 g) oat flour (see Note)

½ teaspoon baking soda

2 teaspoons ground cinnamon

½ teaspoon ground nutmeg

½ teaspoon ground ginger

¼ teaspoon salt

½ cup (60 g) ground flaxseed meal

½ cup (55 g) chopped walnuts, toasted (see Note, page 48)

2 tablespoons (10 g) chia seeds

1 large egg, at room temperature

1 cup packed (225 g) peeled and finely grated or pureed carrots

½ teaspoon vanilla extract

2 tablespoons (30 ml) melted coconut oil or avocado oil

2 to 4 tablespoons (30 to 60 ml) maple syrup, or to taste

½ cup (100 g) semisweet chocolate chips, dairy-free if necessary (optional)

Preheat the oven to 350°F (180°C, or gas mark 4) and line two baking pans with parchment paper or silicone baking sheets.

In a large mixing bowl, add the oats, oat flour, baking soda, cinnamon, nutmeg, ginger, salt, flaxseed meal, walnuts, and chia seeds and stir to combine. Make a well in the middle of the ingredients. Add the egg, carrots, vanilla, and oil to the well and whisk them together, then gently fold the wet ingredients into the dry until thoroughly combined. Add the maple syrup to taste. You can omit this completely for a savory cookie or add up to 4 tablespoons (60 ml) for a sweeter cookie. Stir in the chocolate chips, if desired.

Using a small cookie scoop, scoop the cookie dough onto the pans, placing them about 2 inches (5 cm) apart (there should be about 24 cookies). Flatten each cookie with the back of a spoon or a spatula and bake for 15 to 20 minutes, or until the edges of the cookies are brown and the tops are set. Remove from the oven and let cool on the sheet for about 10 minutes, then transfer to a cooling rack to cool completely. Store in an airtight container in the fridge for 1 week, or freeze for about 1 month (wrap well in plastic and then aluminum foil).

NOTE: To make your own oat flour, place rolled oats in a food processor and process until they resemble a fine crumb.

TIPS:

+ Depending on the moisture in your carrots and the amount of syrup used, there can be some variation in the wetness of the dough. If the dough seems dry and you have trouble getting the cookies to stick together, add 1 additional egg white.

+ I use my food processor to puree the carrots, as I prefer a smooth consistency in the cookies. Be sure to weigh your carrots AFTER processing to ensure the correct amount.

NUTRITION PER SERVING: Serving Size: 28 g, Calories: 90, Total Fat: 4.5 g, Saturated Fat: 1.5 g, Carbohydrates: 9 g, Sugar: 2 g, Sodium: 60 mg, Fiber: 2 g, Protein: 2 g

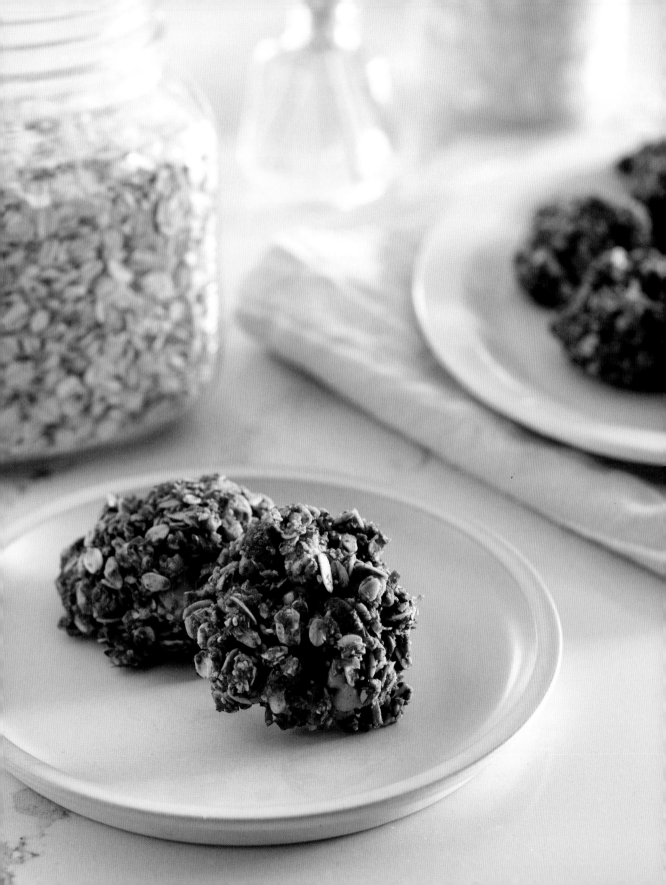

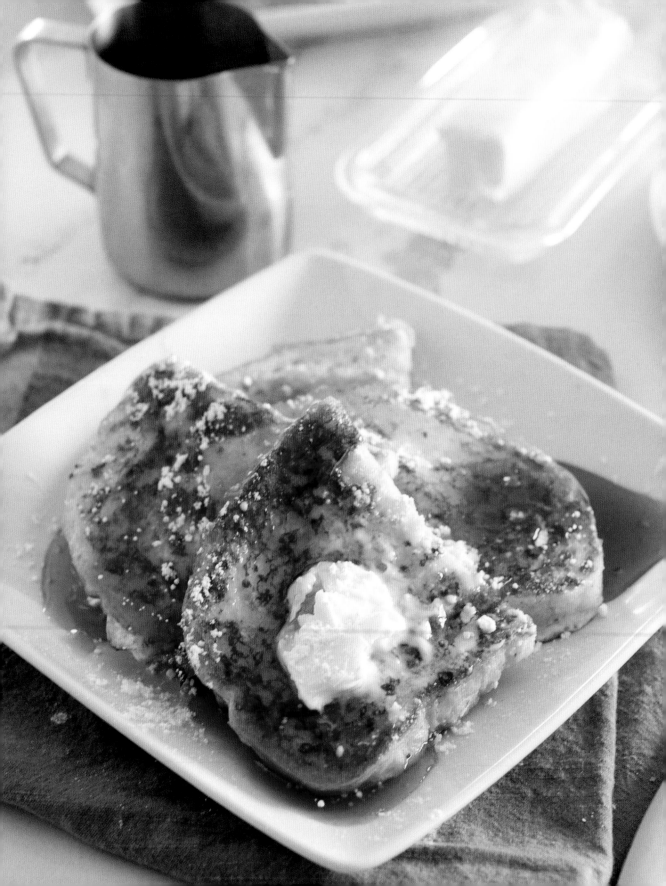

CHAI-SPICED FRENCH TOAST

I first tasted masala chai tea when I traveled in India twenty-five years ago. Using masala chai spice blends in my baked goods brings back those fond memories. This Chai-Spiced French Toast is soft, light, and perfect for breakfast, brunch, or any time of day. I enjoy mine topped with maple syrup and fresh fruit.

Add the eggs, milk, maple extract, and spices to a wide shallow bowl or pie plate and whisk until combined. Add the bread slices to the egg mixture. For a dense bread (like sourdough), let the bread sit for up to 3 minutes on one side, then flip it and let it sit for another 3 minutes to fully absorb the liquid. For a softer bread, simply dip your slices in the egg mixture until saturated but not sopping. Place the dipped bread slices on a separate plate until ready for frying.

Once the bread slices are prepared, heat the oil in a large nonstick skillet over medium heat. Place your egg-soaked bread in the skillet and cook each side until golden brown, about 2 minutes per side. Transfer cooked slices to a plate to keep warm. Serve immediately, along with butter, maple syrup, and confectioners' sugar.

VARIATION: For classic French toast, simply omit the spices for this recipe.

NOTE: I prefer a thick gluten-free bread for this recipe, but any bread will do. Sourdough bread (while not gluten-free) may be low FODMAP if you use white wheat sourdough that has been fermented for 12 hours (see "FODMAP FAQs," page 20). If you tolerate gluten, this is a great alternative.

2 large eggs

½ cup (120 ml) low-FODMAP milk, such as lactose-free or almond milk

1 teaspoon maple extract

½ teaspoon ground cinnamon

¼ teaspoon ground nutmeg

⅛ teaspoon ground cardamom

Pinch of ground cloves

6 slices low-FODMAP, gluten-free, or sourdough bread (see Note)

1 to 2 tablespoons (15 to 30 ml) avocado or canola oil, for frying

NUTRITION PER SERVING: Serving Size: 138 g, Calories: 250, Total Fat: 11 g, Saturated Fat: 2.5 g, Carbohydrates: 30 g, Sugar: 5 g, Sodium: 320 mg, Fiber: 0 g, Protein: 8 g

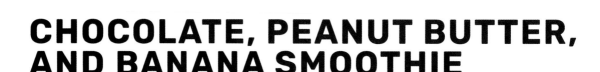

CHOCOLATE, PEANUT BUTTER, AND BANANA SMOOTHIE

This is everyone's favorite smoothie at my house, and for good reason! You can't beat the delicious combination of chocolate, bananas, and peanut butter. I frequently use rolled oats in my smoothies; they improve the texture, fiber, and protein content. For extra energy, you can add some low-FODMAP protein powder too (see Note).

1 cup (235 ml) low-FODMAP milk, such as lactose-free or almond milk

⅓ (35 g) frozen medium ripe banana

2 heaping teaspoons (8 g) cocoa powder

1 tablespoon (15 ml) maple syrup

½ teaspoon vanilla extract

¼ teaspoon ground cinnamon

1 tablespoon (5 g) traditional (old-fashioned) rolled oats

1 tablespoon (15 g) natural peanut butter

½ cup (120 g) ice cubes

1 tablespoon (8 g) low-FODMAP protein powder (optional)

Place all the ingredients in a blender. Blend until creamy, scraping down the sides as necessary. Serve immediately for best results.

TIP: Freeze bananas once they turn brown, and you will always have one ready for your smoothies. No need to waste delicious food!

NOTE: To find a low-FODMAP protein powder, choose one that has been lab-certified, or opt for a product made of brown rice protein, whey protein isolate, or other low-FODMAP ingredients. Be sure to check the label for additives such as inulin and sorbitol.

NUTRITION PER SERVING: Serving Size: 448 g, Calories: 330, Total Fat: 12 g, Saturated Fat: 4 g, Carbohydrates: 46 g, Sugar: 30 g, Sodium: 160 mg, Fiber: 6 g, Protein: 14 g

HOMEMADE CINNAMON CRUNCH BAGEL

I absolutely drool over Panera Cinnamon Crunch Bagels, so I decided to design a shortcut version that we low-FODMAP followers can enjoy. This bagel is also a common request from my son, Jack. It's so easy!

Line a small baking tray for your toaster oven (or air fryer) with aluminum foil. Mix together the cinnamon and both sugars in a small bowl. Place the bagel with the cut-side down on the tray. Spread the bagel liberally with the butter and sprinkle with the cinnamon and sugar mixture to coat. Place in the toaster and lightly toast until the sugar is caramelized and the bagel is done to your liking. Remove and allow to cool slightly so the sugars harden, then spread with your favorite lactose-free cream cheese.

TIP: There are several brands of gluten-free bagels that have low-FODMAP ingredients. I like the texture of Canyon Bakehouse and UDI's.

NOTE: This bagel has a strong cinnamon flavor. If you prefer a little less cinnamon, then opt for ¼ teaspoon instead.

½ teaspoon ground cinnamon

1 teaspoon granulated sugar

½ teaspoon brown sugar

1 low-FODMAP, gluten-free bagel, sliced

1½ teaspoons butter

NUTRITION PER SERVING: Serving Size: 113 g, Calories: 310, Total Fat: 12 g, Saturated Fat: 4.5 g, Carbohydrates: 52 g, Sugar: 9 g, Sodium: 500 mg, Fiber: 4 g, Protein: 4 g

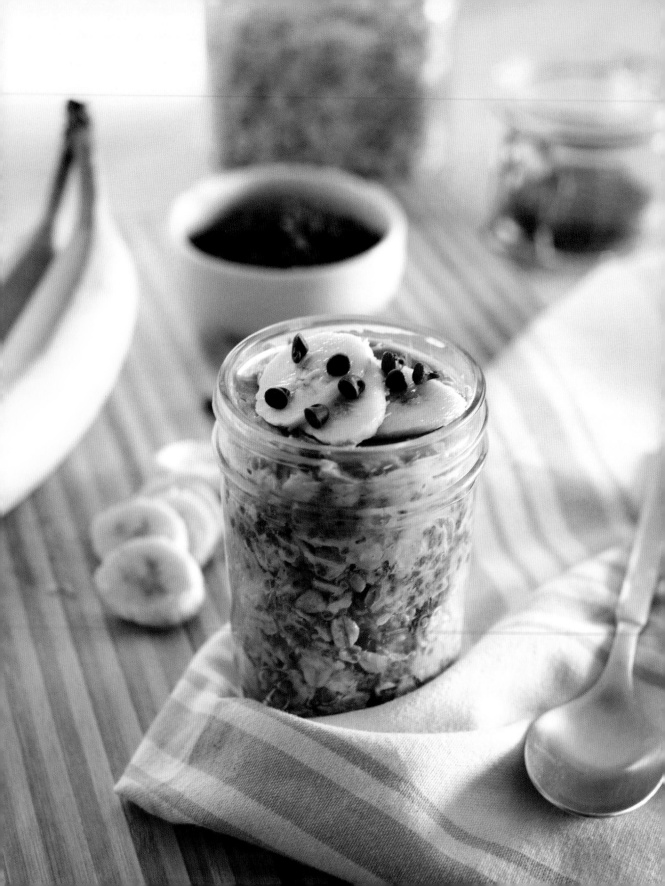

"SPECULOOS COOKIE" TOASTED OVERNIGHT OATS

Overnight oats are a super convenient, grab-and-go breakfast. Toasting the oats adds an extra step, but the flavor difference is completely worth it. Healthy and nourishing, my "speculoos cookie" oats taste like those airplane cookies we all know and love. Enjoy this breakfast cold or warmed in the microwave.

Preheat the oven to 350°F (180°C, or gas mark 4).

Spread the oats on a large rimmed baking sheet and bake for 10 to 15 minutes, until aromatic and toasty. Allow to cool slightly, then add the oats, milk, brown sugar, chia seeds, spices, and salt to a mason jar or covered bowl and stir well to combine. Chill overnight in the refrigerator. Serve topped with almond butter, if desired. May be stored in the refrigerator for 5 days.

VARIATION: Top with chocolate chips, sliced banana, or peanut butter.

½ cup (40 g) traditional (old-fashioned) rolled oats

½ cup (120 ml) low-FODMAP milk, such as lactose-free or almond milk

1 tablespoon (12 g) packed light brown sugar

2 teaspoons chia seeds

½ teaspoon ground cinnamon

⅛ teaspoon ground nutmeg

¹⁄₁₆ teaspoon ground cloves

¹⁄₁₆ teaspoon ground cardamom

Pinch of salt

1 tablespoon (15 g) almond butter (optional)

NUTRITION PER SERVING: Serving Size: 183 g, Calories: 290, Total Fat: 7 g, Saturated Fat: 1.5 g, Carbohydrates: 48 g, Sugar: 19 g, Sodium: 200 mg, Fiber: 7 g, Protein: 10 g

"HUMMINGBIRD" BAKED OATMEAL BARS

Hummingbird cake is a Southern delicacy that originated in Jamaica. It contains pineapple, banana, spices, and pecans. The combination is sublime for baked oats too. FODMAP fact: Canned pineapple "in juice" is low FODMAP in servings of 90 g, while one low-FODMAP serving of fresh pineapple is 140 g.

FOR THE OATMEAL:

2 cups (160 g) traditional (old-fashioned) rolled oats

¼ teaspoon salt

1 teaspoon ground cinnamon

¼ teaspoon ground nutmeg

1 teaspoon baking powder

2 large eggs, at room temperature

½ cup (120 ml) pure maple syrup

½ cup (130 g) chopped fresh pineapple or canned crushed pineapple "in juice," well drained

½ cup (130 g) mashed ripe banana

2 tablespoons (30 ml) melted butter, avocado oil, or melted coconut oil

1½ cups (360 ml) low-FODMAP milk, such as lactose-free or almond milk

1 teaspoon vanilla extract

½ cup (55 g) chopped toasted pecans (see Note), plus more for garnish

FOR THE GLAZE (OPTIONAL):

2 cups (240 g) confectioners' sugar

2 to 4 tablespoons (30 to 60 ml) low-FODMAP milk, such as lactose-free or almond milk

To make the oatmeal: Preheat the oven to 350°F (180°C, or gas mark 4) and grease a 13 x 9-inch (33 x 23 cm) pan with baking spray.

Mix together the rolled oats, salt, spices, and baking powder in a medium bowl. In a large bowl, whisk together the eggs, maple syrup, pineapple, mashed banana, melted butter or oil, milk, and vanilla until well combined. Slowly add the oat mixture and combine by hand. Add the pecans and stir until well incorporated. Pour the mixture into the prepared pan and bake for 35 to 45 minutes, or until set in the middle and golden on the edges. Remove from the oven and allow to cool in the pan on a wire rack.

To make the glaze: Combine the confectioners' sugar and milk in a small bowl until you've reached your desired consistency. Drizzle the glaze over the warm oatmeal and garnish with additional pecans, if desired. Slice the baked oatmeal into 12 bars and serve.

TIP: If you have leftover canned pineapple, you can freeze it for later use (try my Glazed Pineapple Walnut Muffins, page 101).

NOTE: I prefer the flavor of toasted nuts in all my recipes and, fortunately, it's easy to achieve! To toast nuts and seeds, spread them in a single layer on a rimmed baking sheet and place in a 350°F (180°C, or gas mark 4) preheated oven on the middle rack. Bake for 5 to 10 minutes depending on their size. Watch closely so they don't burn. Allow to cool, then use in any recipe as desired.

NUTRITION PER SERVING: Serving Size: 92 g, Calories: 170, Total Fat: 7 g, Saturated Fat: 2 g, Carbohydrates: 25 g, Sugar: 14 g, Sodium: 115 mg, Fiber: 2 g, Protein: 4 g

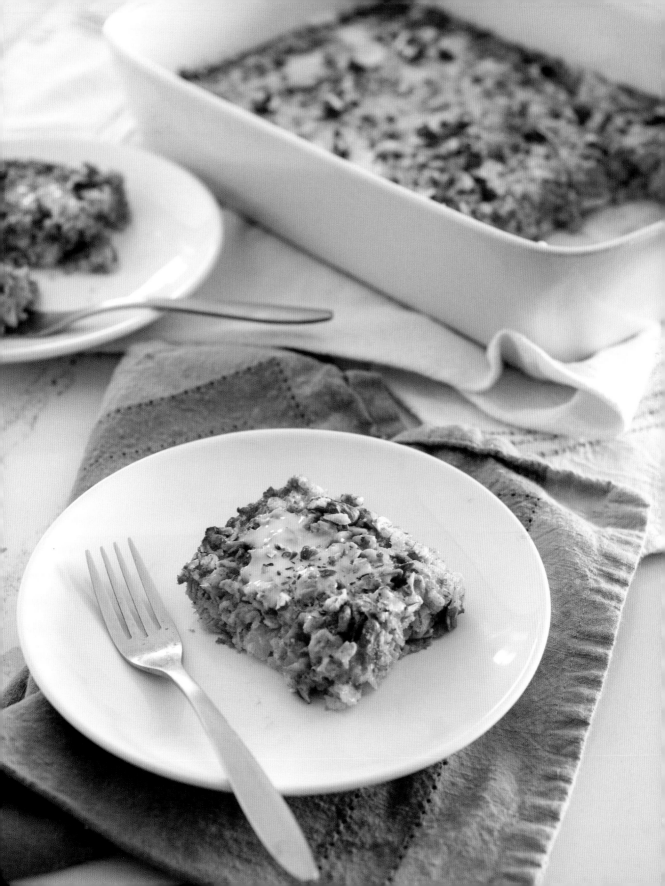

Yield: 4 servings   **Prep time:** 5 minutes   **Cook time:** 5 minutes

DENVER SANDWICH

Also known as a "Western" sandwich, a Denver sandwich consists of a Denver omelet on two slices of toasted bread. My high school cafeteria served Denver sandwiches, and I was recently craving that warm, well-flavored omelet on richly buttered toast. A terrific lunch or supper any day of the week, my version is (almost) as good as my former lunch lady's.

4 large eggs, lightly beaten

2 tablespoons (30 ml) low-FODMAP milk, such as lactose-free or almond milk

½ cup (2 ounces [56 g]) finely chopped precooked deli ham

2 tablespoons (12 g) chopped scallions, green tips only

¼ cup (40 g) finely chopped green bell pepper

⅛ teaspoon salt, plus to taste

⅛ teaspoon freshly ground pepper, plus to taste

1 tablespoon (15 ml) olive or avocado oil

8 slices low-FODMAP, gluten-free bread

Butter or low-FODMAP vegan alternative, to taste

In a large bowl, whisk the eggs and milk until frothy. Stir the ham, scallion tips, green bell peppers, salt, and pepper into the egg. Heat the oil in a 12-inch (30 cm) nonstick skillet over medium heat. Add the egg mixture to the pan and cook, stirring constantly, until the eggs begin to set, 1 to 2 minutes. Use your spatula to gently press and flatten the eggs to about 1 inch (2.5 cm) thick. When sufficiently set to be able to cut, section the omelet into four equal pieces. Flip the pieces and cook to desired doneness, 3 to 4 minutes longer. While the eggs are cooking, toast your bread slices to golden and butter lightly. Serve the eggs between the toasted bread slices while hot.

VARIATION: If you avoid ham, then substitute cubed deli turkey instead.

NUTRITION PER SERVING: Serving Size: 144 g, Calories: 260, Total Fat: 12 g, Saturated Fat: 3 g, Carbohydrates: 27 g, Sugar: 3 g, Sodium: 540 mg, Fiber: 0 g, Protein: 11 g

CHICKEN NOODLE SOUP FOR ONE

Some days I crave soup without wanting to make a whole pot. This is a flavorful recipe for a single serving of warm, nourishing chicken noodle soup. Simple goodness. Dress it up with low-FODMAP crackers or Parmesan cheese.

Add the broth and carrots to a medium pot with a lid and place over medium-high heat. Cover the pot and allow the broth to come to a simmer. Let simmer for 5 minutes, adjusting the heat as necessary, then add the uncooked noodles and chicken. Re-cover and cook according to the package instructions or until the noodles are al dente (5 to 7 minutes). If the broth level looks low, add ¼ to ¾ cup (60 to 180 ml) of filtered water or additional chicken broth. Stir in the infused oil, scallions, salt, and pepper to taste. Serve garnished with fresh parsley.

ADD IT! Toss in some canned, drained, and rinsed corn (50 g) for bonus flavor and texture.

VARIATION: Switch to penne or rotini noodles for a different twist.

NOTE: Since gluten-free pasta tends to get mushy, be sure to cook to al dente. This is Italian for "to the tooth." It means the pasta should still be a tad firm (but not hard) and have a slight resistance when you bite it. Typically, it involves watching your pasta closely and cooking slightly less time than the package recommends.

2 cups (470 ml) low-FODMAP chicken broth or stock, gluten-free if necessary, (see Note, page 61)

1 medium carrot, sliced

1 ounce (28 g) low-FODMAP, gluten-free spaghetti or vermicelli noodles

¾ cup (3 ounces [84 g]) diced or shredded cooked chicken (see Tip, page 53)

1 teaspoon garlic-infused oil

1 scallion, minced, green tips only

¼ teaspoon salt

Pepper

Chopped fresh parsley

NUTRITION PER SERVING: Serving Size: 682 g, Calories: 310, Total Fat: 8 g, Saturated Fat: 1.5 g, Carbohydrates: 30 g, Sugar: 5 g, Sodium: 2610 mg, Fiber: 3 g, Protein: 29 g

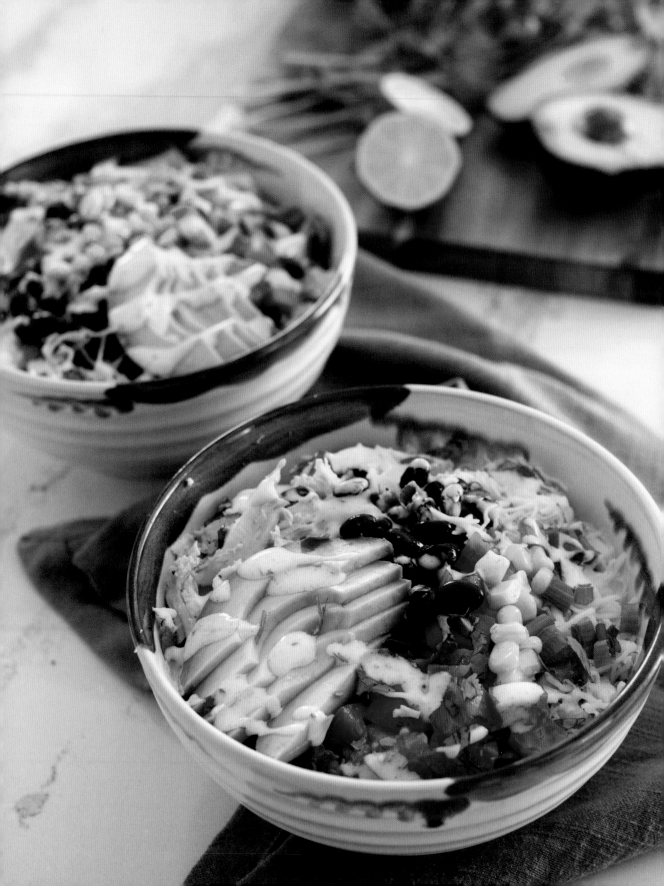

QUINOA POWER BOWL WITH SOUTHWEST DRESSING

My power bowl crushes every fast-food burrito bowl you can buy. Using quinoa gives it extra texture and added protein, and my Southwest dressing is the perfect, zesty topping. Tasty, filling, and so good for you.

To make the dressing: Mix all the dressing ingredients together in a large measuring cup or bowl. Transfer the bowl to the fridge to allow the dressing to chill and the flavors to combine.

To make the quinoa: Combine the rinsed quinoa and chicken broth or water in a medium saucepan and place over medium heat. Let the broth come to a boil and cook until the liquid is mostly absorbed, and the quinoa is cooked through, about 15 minutes. Stir in the olive oil, salt, lime juice, and zest and set aside.

To assemble the bowls: Ladle the quinoa into bowls, then top with the shredded chicken, prepared veggies, cheese, and cilantro. Drizzle with the Southwest dressing and serve. Leftover dressing may be stored in the refrigerator for 5 days.

*Select a mayonnaise with low-FODMAP ingredients (no added onion and garlic), such as Hellmann's.

TIP: I love to precook (bake) chicken breasts and freeze them for a variety of recipes. Place chicken breasts on a lined pan and rub with olive oil, salt, and pepper. Bake at 400°F (200°C, or gas mark 6) for 20 to 30 minutes, depending on their thickness, flipping halfway through cooking. Internal temperature will be 165°F (73°C) when completely cooked.

NOTE: Try the Southwest dressing over a salad topped with cheese, corn, and shredded tortilla chips.

FOR THE DRESSING:

½ cup (120 g) regular or light mayonnaise*

3 tablespoons (45 g) lactose-free sour cream or yogurt

2 tablespoons (30 ml) light corn syrup or maple syrup

2 teaspoons red wine vinegar

1 teaspoon lime juice

½ teaspoon dried cilantro

1 teaspoon chili powder

¼ teaspoon cayenne

¼ teaspoon ground cumin

1 to 2 tablespoons (15 to 30 ml) water (optional, for consistency)

FOR THE QUINOA:

1¼ cups (216 g) uncooked quinoa, rinsed

3 cups (705 ml) low-FODMAP chicken broth, gluten-free if necessary, or water (see Note, page 61)

1 tablespoon (15 ml) olive oil

1 teaspoon salt

Juice and zest of 1 lime

FOR THE BOWL:

3 cups warm or cold, shredded or chopped precooked chicken (about 16 ounces [455 g]) (see Tip)

½ cup (100 g) diced Roma or vine-ripened tomatoes

½ cup (84 g) canned corn, drained and rinsed

½ cup (84 g) canned black beans, drained and rinsed

2 tablespoons (12 g) minced scallions, green tips only

½ avocado (50 g), sliced

¼ cup (30 g) finely shredded white cheddar cheese (optional)

Chopped fresh cilantro

NUTRITION PER SERVING: Serving Size: 506 g, Calories: 640, Total Fat: 40 g, Saturated Fat: 9 g, Carbohydrates: 32 g, Sugar: 12 g, Sodium: 2010 mg, Fiber: 5 g, Protein: 39 g

EASY CAPRESE PANINI

A caprese panini is inspired by the flavors of a caprese salad. Just like its counterpart, it is filled with fresh mozzarella, ripe tomatoes, and aromatic basil, drizzled with balsamic vinegar. FODMAP fact: Mozzarella is naturally low in lactose levels and should be tolerated by most individuals with IBS.

2 slices low-FODMAP, gluten-free or sourdough bread (see "FODMAP FAQs," page 20)

1 tablespoon (15 ml) avocado or olive oil

2 slices (20 g each) fresh mozzarella

2 to 4 (40 g) tomato slices

3 to 4 basil leaves

1 to 2 teaspoons balsamic vinegar

Salt and pepper to taste

Preheat your panini press, or set up a grill pan over medium heat. Brush the outside of one bread slice with oil and place it, oiled-side down, in the panini press or grill pan. Layer the sliced fresh mozzarella, sliced tomato, and basil leaves onto the bread, then carefully drizzle with balsamic vinegar and season lightly with salt and pepper. Brush the other slice of bread with oil and add it to the top of your sandwich, oiled-side up. If using a panini press, close the press and cook until the sandwich is golden. If using a grill pan, place a heavy pan or lid on the sandwich and cook over medium heat until the bottom piece is golden, then flip the sandwich carefully. Grill until the bread is toasted to your preference and the cheese is melted slightly on the edges. Serve immediately.

TIPS:

+ Using fresh mozzarella, basil, red ripe tomatoes, and good-quality balsamic vinegar makes all the difference in this recipe.

+ Store your tomatoes at room temperature (not the fridge) for best results.

NUTRITION PER SERVING: Serving Size: 163 g, Calories: 410, Total Fat: 22 g, Saturated Fat: 6 g, Carbohydrates: 42 g, Sugar: 6 g, Sodium: 330 mg, Fiber: 1 g, Protein: 9 g

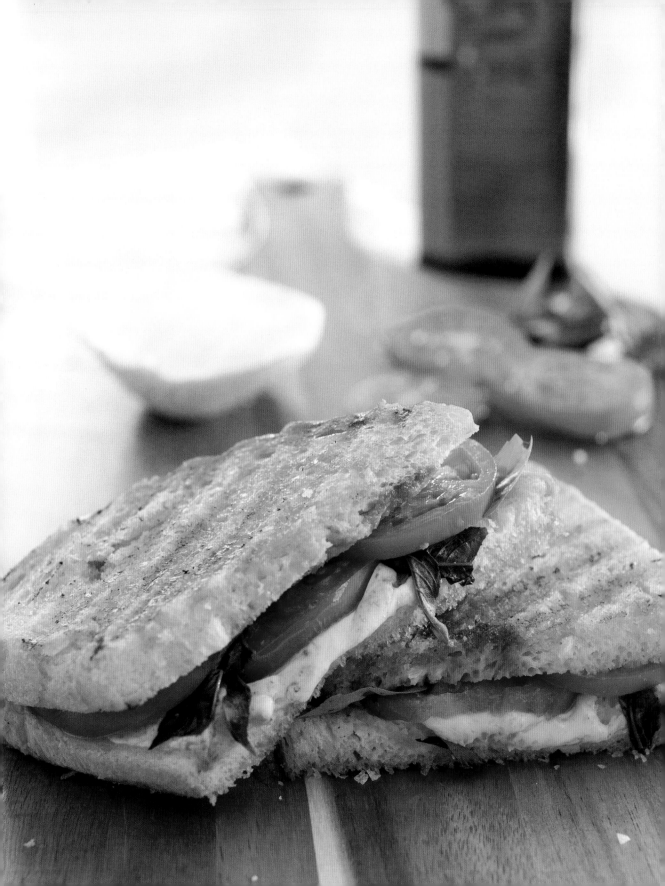

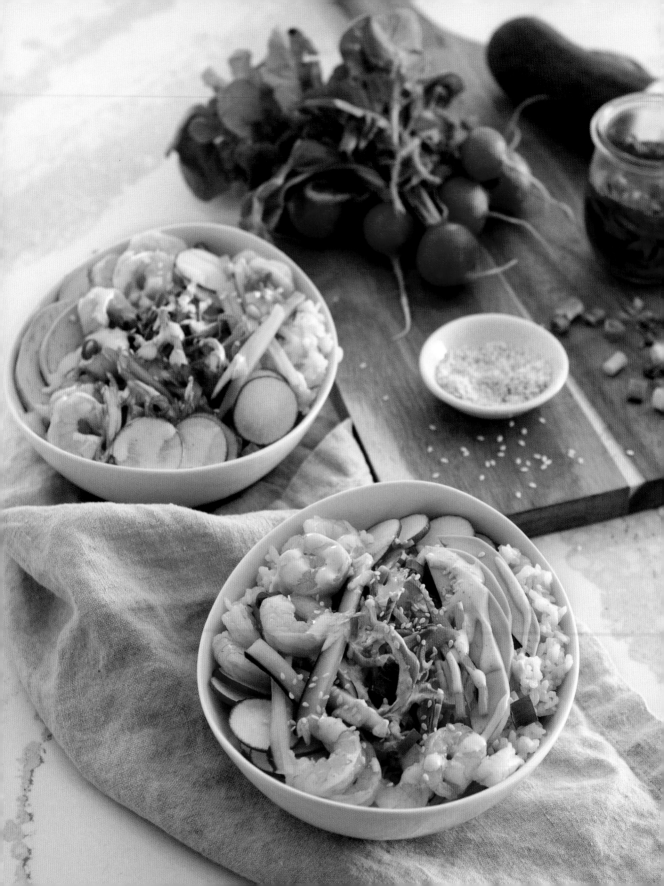

SHRIMP SUSHI BOWL

I am a big fan of sushi and poke bowls and now, with this recipe, I can make them at home, which I love even more! FODMAP facts: FODMAPs were undetected in radishes at servings of 75 g, in common cucumber in servings of 75 g, and in ginger at servings of 5 g. Fermented purple cabbage is low FODMAP in servings up to ½ cup or 75 g.

To make the rice: Cook the sushi rice in a saucepan according to the package instructions. In a small bowl or cup, mix the sugar and rice wine vinegar well, until the sugar dissolves. Once the rice is cooked, remove it from the heat and drizzle the vinegar mixture over the rice. Cover the saucepan and let it sit for 5 minutes.

To make the sriracha mayo: Combine the mayonnaise and sriracha together in a small bowl until smooth.

To assemble the bowl: Scoop rice into two bowls and distribute the shrimp and vegetables evenly between them. Drizzle with soy sauce and sriracha mayo, and top with sesame seeds and scallion tips.

*Select a mayonnaise with low-FODMAP ingredients (no added onion and garlic), such as Hellmann's.

VARIATIONS:

+ You can substitute imitation crab for the shrimp, if desired. Be sure to select a brand that is gluten-free and low FODMAP. Many products contain wheat, sorbitol, pea protein, and high-fructose syrup, so be sure to check your labels (see "How to Read Labels," page 26).

+ Try this with some edamame (90 g per serving), chopped cherry tomatoes (45 g per serving), and crushed peanuts for a different, equally delicious option.

FOR THE RICE:

¾ cup (150 g) uncooked sushi rice, rinsed well

1 teaspoon sugar

2 tablespoons (30 ml) rice wine vinegar

FOR THE SRIRACHA MAYO:

2 tablespoons (30 g) mayonnaise*

1 to 2 teaspoons sriracha, to taste

FOR THE BOWL:

8 ounces (227 g) precooked and deveined shrimp, tails off

1 large carrot, sliced into ribbons or strips

4 tablespoons (35 g) pickled (fermented) red cabbage

4 radishes (60 g), sliced

1-inch (2.5 cm) piece of fresh ginger root, finely sliced, or 1 tablespoon pickled, sliced ginger

½ common cucumber (80 g), sliced into ribbons or strips

¼ to ½ ripe avocado (50 g), sliced

2 to 4 tablespoons (30 to 40 ml) soy sauce, gluten-free if necessary

1 teaspoon toasted sesame seeds

1 tablespoon (6 g) minced scallions, green tips only

NUTRITION PER SERVING: Serving Size: 401 g, Calories: 710, Total Fat: 28 g, Saturated Fat: 4.5 g, Carbohydrates: 88 g, Sugar: 9 g, Sodium: 1770 mg, Fiber: 6 g, Protein: 25 g

CHICKEN CLUB RANCH PASTA SALAD

A classic. There is nothing in this salad I don't love. Take it to a picnic or potluck, and it will vanish in minutes. As a bonus, you can also enjoy the ranch dressing over a garden salad, as a veggie dip, or for dunking potato chips.

FOR RANCH DRESSING:

2 teaspoons garlic-infused oil

¾ cup (180 g) mayonnaise*

3 tablespoons (45 g) lactose-free sour cream

2 teaspoons dried chives

1 teaspoon dried dill

1 teaspoon dried parsley

1 tablespoon (6 g) minced scallions, green tips only

1 teaspoon fresh lemon juice

Pinch of kosher salt, plus more to taste

FOR THE SALAD:

8 ounces (227 g) uncooked low-FODMAP, gluten-free rotini, penne, or elbow macaroni

1 teaspoon olive oil

8 slices (8 ounces [227 g]) cooked, chopped bacon or turkey bacon

2 cups (250 g) cooked, chopped chicken, cold (see Tip, page 53)

150 g avocado, diced (this may be 1 to 2 avocados, depending on size)

1 large tomato (130 g), diced

1 cup (75 g) canned corn, drained and rinsed

¾ cup (100 g) cubed or shredded Cheddar cheese

To make the dressing: Combine all the dressing ingredients in a large bowl or measuring cup. Set this aside in the refrigerator for later.

To make the salad: In a large saucepan, cook the pasta according to the package directions (about 7 minutes; see Tip). Rinse the pasta under cold water and drain well. Add the pasta to a large serving bowl and toss with the olive oil to keep the noodles from sticking together. Add the remaining ingredients, except the dressing, to the bowl and toss to combine. Add as much dressing as you'd like and toss to coat or serve the salad as is, with the dressing on the side. May be served warm or cold. Leftover dressing may be stored in the refrigerator for 5 days.

*Select a mayonnaise with low-FODMAP ingredients (no added onion and garlic), such as Hellmann's.

VARIATION: To make this even more delicious, use fresh herbs to make the ranch dressing. Substitute 2 tablespoons (10 g) chopped fresh chives, 1 tablespoon (5 g) chopped fresh dill, and 1 tablespoon (4 g) chopped fresh parsley for their dried counterparts.

TIP: For a cold pasta salad, I recommend cooking your gluten-free pasta a little longer than you would if you were cooking it for a soup. Whereas the noodles will get mushy in a sauce or broth, they can end up chewy and hard when chilled (particularly if your gluten-free pasta contains a combination of corn and rice flours). Experiment with your product to see how you prefer your pasta.

NUTRITION PER SERVING: Serving Size: 235 g, Calories: 750, Total Fat: 54 g, Saturated Fat: 15 g, Carbohydrates: 36 g, Sugar: 2 g, Sodium: 1150 mg, Fiber: 2 g, Protein: 32 g

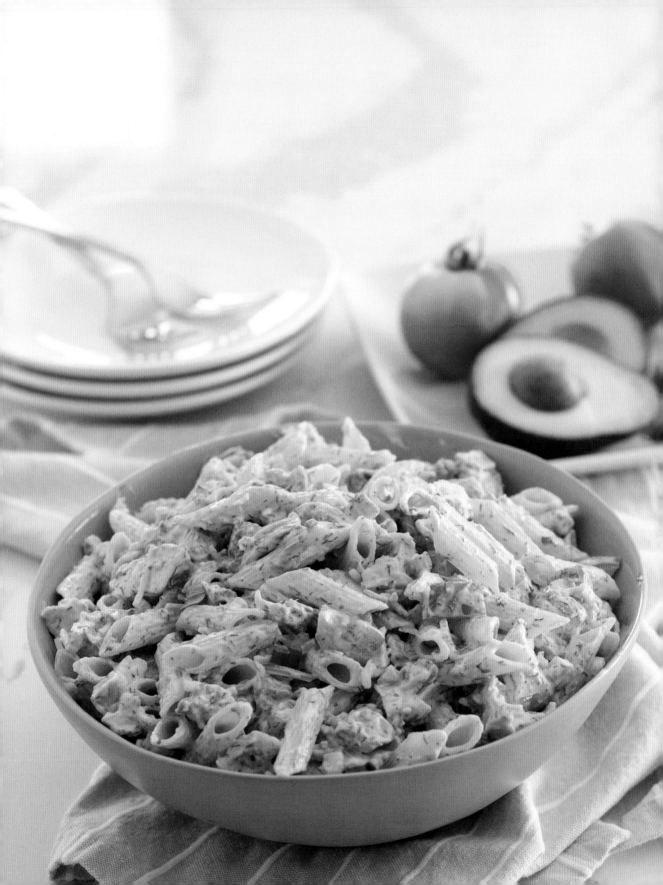

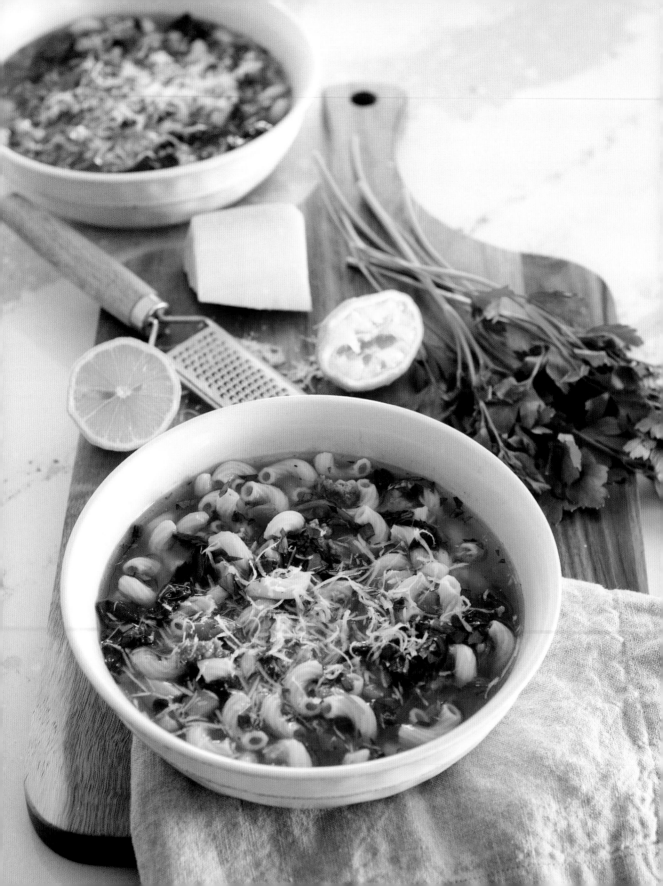

HEARTY TURKEY MINESTRONE SOUP

This turkey minestrone soup is packed with amazing ingredients and makes enough to satisfy your whole family. I prefer a thick consistency to my soup, but you can thin out the broth according to your preference. FODMAP fact: Only trace FODMAPs are found in kale, so you may enjoy this vegetable as much as you like.

In a large 5- to 6-quart (4.5 to 5.4 L) saucepan or Dutch oven, brown the turkey over medium heat for 8 to 10 minutes, breaking it into smaller pieces as it browns. Once cooked, add the carrots, tomatoes, 4 cups (940 ml) of vegetable broth, water, tomato paste, and dried herbs and stir well. Cover the pan and cook for about 5 minutes to soften the carrots. Remove the lid, add the squash and gluten-free pasta, and season with salt and pepper. Cover again and simmer for about 10 minutes, then add the spinach or kale, infused oil, and up to 2 additional cups (470 ml) of vegetable broth, until the soup reaches your desired consistency. Lower the heat as necessary so the soup is sitting at a gentle simmer. Simmer for 8 minutes or until the pasta is cooked to al dente and the greens are tender. Taste the broth and add seasonings if desired. Remove the pot from the heat and stir in the lemon juice. Serve in bowls garnished with grated Parmesan and fresh parsley, if desired.

*Make sure there is no added onion or garlic in your diced canned tomatoes and tomato paste.

TIP: To make ahead, cook your pasta in a separate pot to al dente, then add it to the soup just before serving. This prevents the pasta from getting mushy over time.

NOTE: Finding a low-FODMAP chicken, beef, or vegan broth/soup base can be challenging. Most products have added onion and garlic, so be savvy in selecting. I have recipes on my website to make these from scratch; for an easier option you can shop for lab-certified low-FODMAP soup bases at www.rachelpaulsfood.com.

1 pound (455 g) uncooked ground turkey (or ground chicken)

3 medium carrots (200 g), chopped

1 (14-ounce [392 g]) can diced tomatoes, with their liquid*

4 cups (940 ml) low-FODMAP vegetable broth or stock, plus 2 cups (470 ml) as desired, divided, gluten-free if necessary (see Note)

2 cups (470 ml) water

½ cup (120 g) tomato paste*

½ teaspoon dried oregano

½ teaspoon dried thyme

1 cup (150 g) chopped yellow summer squash

1 cup (8 ounces [227 g]) uncooked low-FODMAP, gluten-free ditalini, fusilli, or elbow macaroni

Salt and pepper to taste

¾ cup (25 g) baby spinach or chopped kale, torn

1 tablespoon (15 ml) onion- or shallot-infused oil

2 teaspoons freshly squeezed lemon juice

¼ cup (25 g) freshly grated Parmesan cheese, for garnish (optional)

Chopped fresh parsley, for garnish (optional)

NUTRITION PER SERVING: Serving Size: 422 g, Calories: 280, Total Fat: 8 g, Saturated Fat: 2 g, Carbohydrates: 32 g, Sugar: 6 g, Sodium: 830 mg, Fiber: 3 g, Protein: 19 g

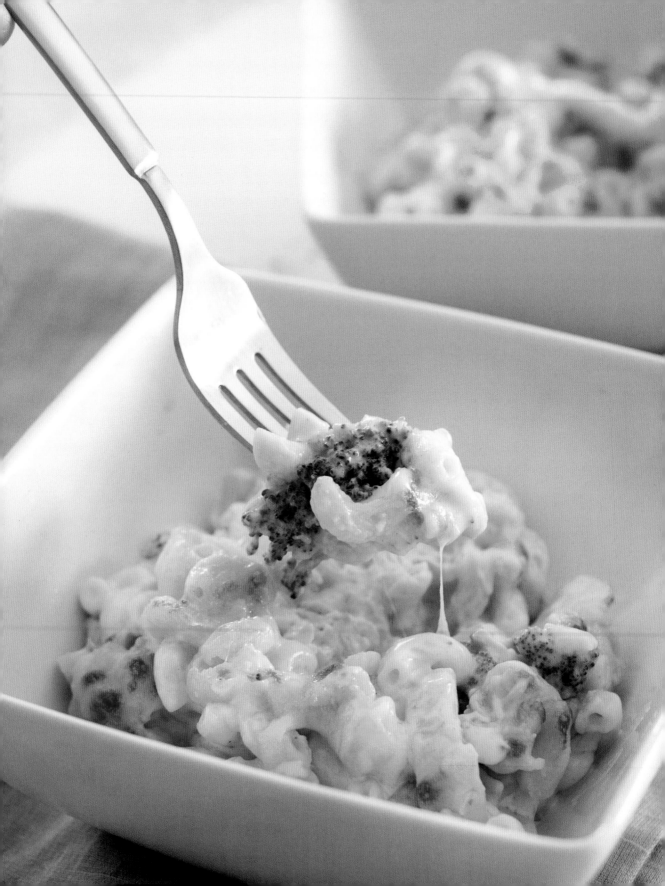

THE BEST MACARONI AND CHEESE WITH VEGETABLES

My macaroni and cheese is a great way to get your kids to eat their veggies. It's so creamy, rich, and packed with real cheese flavor. FODMAP fact: Cheese is naturally low in lactose. Although both Monash and FODMAP Friendly apps list a low-FODMAP serving of 40 g for Cheddar cheese, the maximum portion that may be consumed from a FODMAP standpoint is 462 g. However, because excessive fat can trigger gut irritation, stick to the recommended serving size suggested for this recipe.

Preheat the oven broiler on high. Fill a large oven-safe saucepan or 6-quart (5.4 L) Dutch oven three-fourths full with water and bring it to a boil over high heat. Add the macaroni and boil for 5 to 7 minutes, or until al dente (do not overcook).

While the macaroni is cooking, warm the oil in a 10-inch (25 cm) skillet over medium heat. Add the broccoli and squash to the pan and sprinkle with salt. Sauté the vegetables for 5 to 7 minutes, until softened but still crisp. Remove from the heat.

When the pasta is al dente, drain it and set it aside (do not rinse; you want the pasta to stay warm). Return the saucepan or Dutch oven to the stove, turn the heat to medium, and add the butter. Once the butter is melted, stir in the flour. Slowly add the milk, followed by the half-and-half, stirring continuously. Bring the sauce to a boil, then lower the heat to a simmer and stir for 2 minutes, allowing it to thicken. Add 2 cups (226 g) of the grated cheese, salt, and pepper and stir until the cheese is completely melted and incorporated into the sauce. Add the drained macaroni and vegetables and mix gently to combine well. Top with the remaining 1 cup (113 g) of grated cheese and place the saucepan in the oven to broil for 2 to 3 minutes, until the cheese melts. Let cool slightly, then serve immediately.

VARIATION: Try zucchini and carrots instead of broccoli and summer squash.

TIP: Since gluten-free pasta gets mushy with time, this macaroni is best enjoyed immediately.

1 pound (455 g) uncooked low-FODMAP, gluten-free elbow macaroni

1 teaspoon olive oil

1 cup (100 g) chopped broccoli heads

1 cup (150 g) cubed or quartered into crescents yellow summer squash

1 teaspoon salt, plus more for sprinkling

½ cup (112 g) unsalted butter

⅓ cup (40 g) low-FODMAP, gluten-free flour

1 cup (235 ml) lactose-free whole milk, such as lactose-free or almond milk

2 cups (470 ml) lactose-free half-and-half

3 cups (about 340 g) freshly shredded cheese, such as sharp Cheddar or Colby Jack, divided

½ teaspoon black pepper

NUTRITION PER SERVING: Serving Size: 241 g, Calories: 600, Total Fat: 36 g, Saturated Fat: 20 g, Carbohydrates: 51 g, Sugar: 4 g, Sodium: 610 mg, Fiber: 1 g, Protein: 18 g

BROWN SUGAR-GLAZED MEATLOAF

You can never go wrong with this suppertime classic. My recipe makes for a tender, juicy meatloaf, covered with a tangy, sweet glaze. Serve it with mashed potatoes and carrots or a side salad.

FOR THE BROWN SUGAR GLAZE:

7 tablespoons (105 g) canned tomato paste*

5 tablespoons (75 ml) water or low-FODMAP beef broth, gluten-free if necessary (see Note, page 61)

1 tablespoon (15 ml) Worcestershire sauce (gluten-free if necessary)

1 teaspoon white vinegar (gluten-free if necessary)

½ cup (100 g) lightly packed brown sugar

¼ teaspoon mustard powder

¼ teaspoon salt

FOR THE MEATLOAF:

1 teaspoon garlic-infused oil

1 pound (455 g) lean ground beef

1 large egg

½ cup (60 g) low-FODMAP, gluten-free bread crumbs

½ teaspoon ground black pepper

¼ teaspoon ground ginger

1 teaspoon salt

1 tablespoon (6 g) chopped scallions, green tips only

2 to 4 tablespoons (30 to 60 ml) low-FODMAP milk, such as lactose-free or almond milk

Preheat the oven to 350°F (180°C, or gas mark 4) and place a rack in the center of the oven.

To make the glaze: Place all the glaze ingredients in a medium bowl and stir until well combined.

To make the meatloaf: In a separate medium bowl, mix all the meatloaf ingredients except the milk with your hands or a wooden spoon. Add the milk a little at a time until the mixture reaches a consistency that can be easily shaped into a loaf (be careful not to overhandle the meat). Place the meatloaf in a 9 x 5-inch (23 x 13 cm) loaf pan and brush all over with the glaze. Bake, uncovered, for 55 minutes, or until an instant-read meat thermometer inserted into the thickest part of the loaf reads at least 160°F (70°C). Remove from the oven and allow to stand for 5 to 10 minutes, then slice and serve.

*Make sure there is no added onion or garlic in the tomato paste.

ADD IT! If you like a little texture in your meatloaf, then finely chop about ¼ cup (50 g) each of green pepper and/or carrots and add these to the meat mixture. You may not need milk in this instance due to the added moisture from the vegetables.

NUTRITION PER SERVING: Serving Size: 229 g, Calories: 420, Total Fat: 16 g, Saturated Fat: 6 g, Carbohydrates: 42 g, Sugar: 29 g, Sodium: 950 mg, Fiber: 2 g, Protein: 27 g

SAVORY BACON-WRAPPED SCALLOPS

Bacon-wrapped scallops are an elegant choice for an appetizer or a main course. About four scallops make up one hearty serving. For a savory-sweet version of this recipe, see the variation. FODMAP fact: Bacon is low FODMAP in servings of two strips. However, because it is high in fat, limit your intake to reduce IBS symptoms.

Preheat the oven to 425°F (220°C, or gas mark 7) and place a rack in the center of the oven. Line a baking sheet with parchment paper and set aside.

Cut the bacon into strips long enough to wrap around the sides of a scallop once (you want there to be enough bacon to completely encircle the scallop, but not so much that the bacon doesn't cook). Wrap the bacon strips around the outside of the scallops, leaving the tops and bottoms uncovered, and secure each with a toothpick. Place the wrapped scallops on the prepared baking sheet with 1 to 2 inches (2.5 to 5 cm) of space between each scallop. Sprinkle a few drops of olive oil over each of the scallops and season with salt and pepper. Bake for 12 to 17 minutes, until the scallops are tender and opaque and the bacon is cooked through (the bacon will be cooked, but not crisp).

VARIATION: If you want a hint of sweetness on your scallops (my favorite), make a glaze by mixing 3 tablespoons (45 g) brown sugar and 1 teaspoon powdered ginger in a bowl and sprinkle it over each scallop prior to baking. After 7 minutes, remove the pan from the oven, turn the scallops over, and sprinkle again. Finish cooking per the directions.

NOTES:

+ Scallops are easy to overcook (they become rubbery), so pay attention to their doneness. Select scallops of uniform size to ensure they cook evenly, keeping in mind that larger scallops will be more tender once cooked.

+ In this recipe, the bacon will be cooked but still soft. If you prefer crisp bacon, then precook it partially in the microwave. Lay half strips of bacon between paper towels and heat until just curling at the edges (about 2 minutes) before wrapping scallops.

8 slices regular bacon

16 sea scallops (about 1 pound [455 g]), patted dry

2 tablespoons (30 ml) olive oil

Salt and pepper to taste

NUTRITION PER SERVING: Serving Size: 177 g, Calories: 370, Total Fat: 30 g, Saturated Fat: 9 g, Carbohydrates: 4 g, Sugar: 1 g, Sodium: 820 mg, Fiber: 0 g, Protein: 21 g

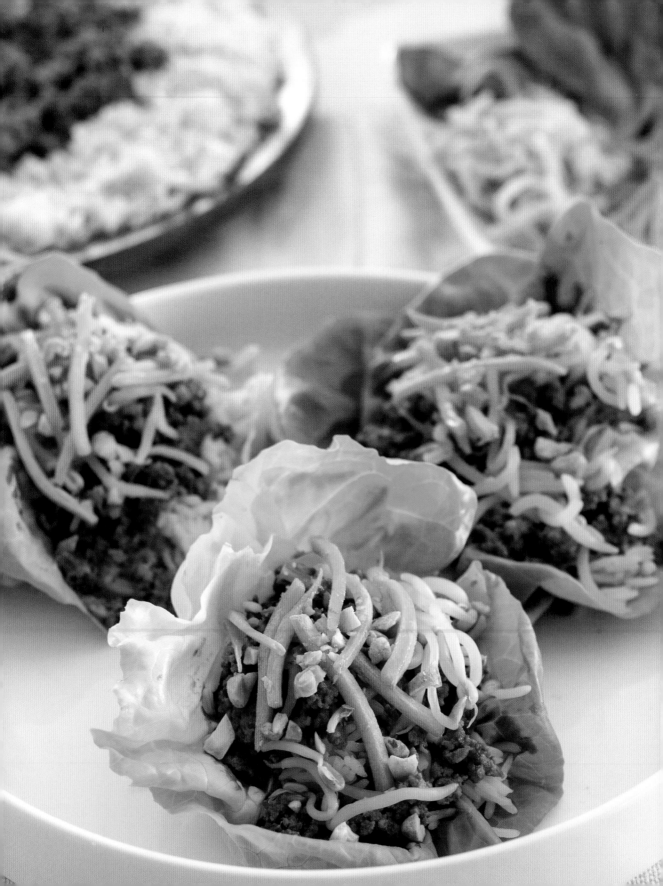

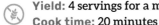
"HARVEST IN SNOW" ASIAN LETTUCE WRAPS

This dish was inspired by a similar meal at one of my favorite childhood Chinese restaurants. The restaurant is no longer open, but my memory of this meal lives on. I bet you will love it as much as I do. FODMAP fact: Oyster mushrooms are low FODMAP in 75-gram servings; do not substitute other mushrooms for this recipe.

To make the sauce: Mix the ingredients for the sauce in a small bowl and set aside.

To make the marinade: In a medium bowl, combine all the marinade ingredients.

To make the filling: Add the ground chicken and ground pork to the bowl with the marinade and use your hands to lightly mix everything together.

Add the water to a medium pot over medium-high heat and bring to a boil. When the water is boiling, add the rice and boil, uncovered, for about 8 minutes, or until tender. Drain any excess water, if necessary, then cover the pot and allow the rice to sit for about 10 minutes. Fluff with a fork once completed cooking.

While the rice is cooking, heat 1 tablespoon (15 ml) of the oil in a skillet and brown the meat mixture over medium heat until well cooked, 5 to 7 minutes, breaking the meat into pieces as it browns. Drain the meat and transfer to a plate to keep warm. Add the remaining 1 tablespoon (15 ml) of oil to the same skillet, then add the mushrooms, water chestnuts, and scallions. Stir-fry the veggies for about a minute, then add the meat back to the skillet and cover with the sauce. Stir-fry until everything is well coated with sauce and heated through. Remove from the heat.

Continued on page 70

FOR THE SAUCE:

1 tablespoon (15 ml) light soy sauce, gluten-free if necessary

¼ teaspoon salt

½ teaspoon sugar

¼ teaspoon black pepper

1 teaspoon sesame oil

FOR THE MARINADE:

3 large egg yolks

1 tablespoon (15 ml) light soy sauce, gluten-free if necessary

1 tablespoon (15 ml) water

1 tablespoon (8 g) cornstarch

¼ teaspoon black pepper

1 teaspoon sesame oil

continued from page 69

FOR THE FILLING:

8 ounces (225 g) ground chicken or turkey

8 ounces (225 g) ground pork or beef

2½ cups (590 ml) water

1½ cups (240 g) uncooked jasmine rice, rinsed

2 tablespoons (30 ml) canola or avocado oil, divided

¼ cup (20 g) chopped oyster mushrooms

½ cup (75 g) chopped canned water chestnuts

2 tablespoons (12 g) chopped scallions, green tips only

FOR SERVING:

1 to 2 heads leaf lettuce, cleaned and separated (about 8 leaves total)

Low-FODMAP, gluten-free hoisin sauce (see Tip)

Optional toppings: bean sprouts, shredded carrot, chopped peanuts

To serve, spread the rice onto a large serving platter ("snow"), and add the meat on top ("harvest"). To eat, take a leaf of lettuce and spread it with a small amount of hoisin sauce, then scoop the rice and meat mixture onto the lettuce leaf, add any optional toppings, and fold to enjoy.

TIP: You can make your own hoisin sauce using my low-FODMAP, gluten-free, vegan recipe, which can be found on my website at www.rachelpaulsfood.com. If using a store-bought brand, San-J is FODMAP Friendly certified and gluten-free.

NUTRITION PER SERVING: Serving Size: 431 g, Calories: 640, Total Fat: 30 g, Saturated Fat: 8 g, Carbohydrates: 57 g, Sugar: 3 g, Sodium: 710 mg, Fiber: 2 g, Protein: 32 g

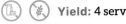
SHEET PAN ORANGE CHICKEN WITH BROCCOLI

This Asian-inspired sheet pan chicken dinner will blow you away. Tender morsels of chicken, slightly crispy from pan baking, drenched in a fresh and zesty orange sauce—what's not to love? Serve it over rice to soak up all that extra sauce.

To make the chicken: Preheat the oven to 450°F (230°C, or gas mark 8) and place a rack in the center of the oven. Line a rimmed baking sheet with aluminum foil and spray with baking spray.

Set up a dredging station with two medium bowls. Whisk the egg in one bowl and add the low-FODMAP flour to the other. Gently toss the chicken pieces, one by one, in the egg, then lightly dredge in the flour. Lay each piece on one side of your baking sheet. Once all the chicken is coated, drizzle with 1 tablespoon (15 ml) of each of the infused oils and ½ tablespoon (7.5 ml) of the sesame oil.

Lay your broccoli and scallion tips on the other side of the baking sheet and toss with the remaining 1 tablespoon (15 ml) of each infused oil and the remaining ½ tablespoon (7.5 ml) of sesame oil. Sprinkle everything with the salt and pepper. Transfer the baking sheet to the oven and bake for 12 minutes, then remove from the oven to toss the veggies and flip the chicken pieces. Return to the oven for another 3 to 8 minutes, until the veggies are cooked and the chicken has reached an internal temperature of 165°F (73°C) when tested with a meat thermometer.

To make the sauce: In a large skillet or saucepan (big enough for your chicken and broccoli), combine the orange zest, orange juice, soy sauce, corn syrup, brown sugar, rice vinegar, ginger, and red pepper flakes, if using. Set the pan over medium-high heat and bring the sauce to a boil. Boil for 5 to 8 minutes, until the sauce thickens and reduces by about one-third. If desired, stir in the cornstarch slurry; this will make the sauce even thicker. Once the sauce is your desired consistency, remove from the heat and cover to keep warm.

Continued on page 72

FOR THE CHICKEN:

1 large egg, at room temperature

⅓ cup (40 g) low-FODMAP, gluten-free flour

1½ pounds (680 g) boneless, skinless chicken breasts, cut into 2-inch (5 cm) cubes

2 tablespoons (30 ml) garlic-infused oil, divided

2 tablespoons (30 ml) onion- or shallot-infused oil, divided

1 tablespoon (15 ml) toasted sesame oil, divided

3 cups (300 g) broccoli florets

3 scallions, green tips only, cut into ½-inch (1.3 cm) slices

½ teaspoon kosher salt, plus more to taste

½ teaspoon black pepper, plus more to taste

continued from page 71

FOR THE ORANGE SAUCE:

Zest and juice of 1 large orange
(¼ to ⅓ cup [60 to 80 ml]),
freshly squeezed

¼ cup (60 ml) light soy sauce,
gluten-free if necessary

6 tablespoons (90 ml) light
corn syrup

¼ cup (50 g) brown sugar

3 tablespoons (45 ml) rice wine
vinegar or apple cider vinegar

1 tablespoon (6 g) freshly
grated ginger

1 teaspoon crushed red pepper
flakes, or to taste (optional)

2 tablespoons (16 g) cornstarch
dissolved in ¼ cup (60 ml) water
(optional)

FOR SERVING:

Steamed rice

Chopped scallions, green tips only

Toasted sesame seeds

When the chicken and broccoli are fully cooked, remove the sheet from the oven and immediately add the meat and veggies to the sauce. Toss everything together until the chicken and broccoli are thoroughly coated. Remove from the heat and serve over bowls of rice, garnished with green scallion tips and sesame seeds.

TIP: If you like a very potent orange flavor, then add ¼ teaspoon of orange extract or flavoring.

NOTE: Fresh orange juice and zest make all the difference in this recipe. Do not substitute canned or bottled juice, as it has not been tested for FODMAP content.

NUTRITION PER SERVING: Serving Size: 388 g, Calories: 590, Total Fat: 22 g, Saturated Fat: 3.5 g, Carbohydrates: 58 g, Sugar: 43 g, Sodium: 940 mg, Fiber: 2 g, Protein: 43 g

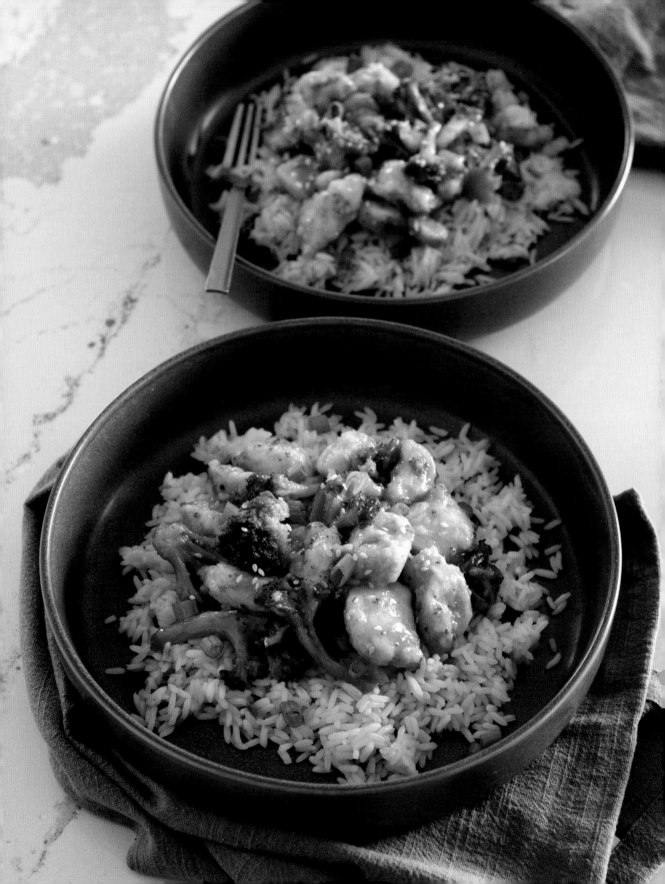

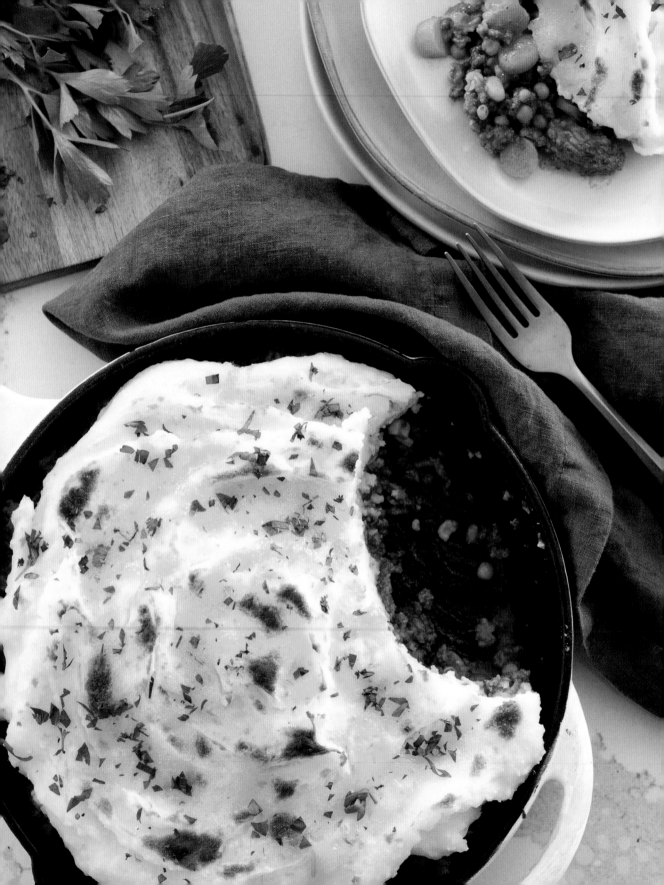

SKILLET COTTAGE PIE

I recently learned the difference between a "cottage pie" and a "shepherd's pie." It's dictated by the type of meat used in the recipe. While a shepherd's pie is made with lamb, a cottage pie uses beef instead. This cottage pie is a snap to make, incorporating leftover mashed potatoes and one skillet for easy cleanup.

Preheat the oven to 375°F (190°C, or gas mark 5).

Heat the oil in an 11-inch (27 cm) oven-safe skillet (such as cast iron) over medium-high heat, then add the ground beef. Cook the beef until browned, 8 to 10 minutes, breaking the meat into smaller pieces to ensure it cooks thoroughly. Add the salt to the beef while it is browning, and stir into the meat. Once the beef is cooked, transfer to a plate and set aside. Drain any grease from the skillet and return it to the stove.

Add the carrots and celery to the skillet and adjust the heat to medium. Cook, stirring occasionally, for 2 to 3 minutes, then add the tomato paste and oregano and cook for another 3 minutes. Stir in the beef broth, Worcestershire sauce, and black pepper. Mix in the cooked beef, peas, and corn. Simmer for a few minutes, then add both infused oils. Taste, and adjust the seasonings as desired.

Spoon the prepared mashed potatoes over the beef and smooth out the top, then sprinkle with the Parmesan cheese. Transfer the cottage pie to the oven and bake for 40 to 45 minutes, until the potatoes are browned and slightly crisp on top. Let cool for 5 to 10 minutes, then sprinkle with the minced fresh parsley before serving.

*Make sure there is no added onion or garlic in the tomato paste.

VARIATION: To make this a "shepherd's pie," use lamb instead of beef.

NOTE: If you don't have premade mashed potatoes, then you will need 5 or 6 russet potatoes for this dish. I have a great recipe for low-FODMAP, gluten-free, vegan mashed potatoes at www.rachelpaulsfood.com.

1 tablespoon (15 ml) avocado or canola oil

2 pounds (910 g) lean ground beef

1 teaspoon kosher salt, plus more to taste

3 carrots (200 g), peeled and diced or chopped

1 medium celery stalk (40 g), chopped

6 tablespoons (90 g) tomato paste*

1½ teaspoons dried oregano

1 cup (235 ml) low-FODMAP beef stock or broth, gluten-free if necessary (see Note, page 61)

1 teaspoon Worcestershire sauce, gluten-free if necessary

½ teaspoon black pepper, plus more to taste

½ cup (90 g) canned peas, rinsed and drained

½ cup (90 g) canned corn, rinsed and drained

1 tablespoon (15 ml) garlic-infused oil

1 tablespoon (15 ml) onion- or shallot-infused oil

4 cups (2 pounds [910 g]) prepared mashed potatoes

¼ cup (30 g) shredded Parmesan cheese or ⅓ cup (40 g) shredded Cheddar cheese

Minced fresh parsley, for garnish

NUTRITION PER SERVING: Serving Size: 332 g, Calories: 400, Total Fat: 21 g, Saturated Fat: 7 g, Carbohydrates: 25 g, Sugar: 4 g, Sodium: 870 mg, Fiber: 2 g, Protein: 28 g

LEMON PARMESAN CHICKEN PICCATA

Chicken piccata is my favorite gourmet meal to serve at a dinner party. This recipe incorporates some extra special touches: a Parmesan breading, creamy sauce, and fresh herbs. It is decadent heaven.

FOR THE CHICKEN:

4 boneless, skinless chicken breasts (1½ pounds [680 g] total)

1 teaspoon salt

½ teaspoon black pepper

2 tablespoons (16 g) low-FODMAP, gluten-free flour

2 tablespoons (12 g) finely grated fresh Parmesan cheese

FOR THE SAUCE:

2 tablespoons (30 ml) garlic-infused oil, divided

1¼ cups (295 ml) low-FODMAP chicken broth or stock, gluten-free if necessary (see Note, page 61)

½ cup (120 ml) heavy cream or canned coconut cream

⅓ cup (35 g) finely grated fresh Parmesan cheese

4 tablespoons (32 g) capers, divided

2 to 3 tablespoons (30 to 45 ml) fresh lemon juice

2 tablespoons (8 g) chopped fresh parsley

Salt and pepper to taste

To make the chicken: Lay the chicken breasts between two pieces of plastic wrap or parchment paper. Using a mallet, firmly pound them until they're about ½ inch (1.3 cm) thick. Remove the plastic wrap and season the chicken with the salt and pepper. Combine the flour and Parmesan cheese in a shallow bowl. Dredge each piece of chicken in the flour mixture and set it aside on a plate or chopping board.

To make the sauce: Pour 1 tablespoon (15 ml) of the infused oil into a large skillet over medium-high heat. Fry the chicken until the breading is golden brown and a meat thermometer inserted into the thickest part of the meat registers 160°F (70°C), 3 to 4 minutes per side, depending on the thickness of your chicken. Transfer the chicken to a warm plate and set aside.

Lower the heat to medium-low and add the remaining 1 tablespoon (15 ml) of infused oil, chicken broth, and cream. Bring the sauce to a gentle simmer, then add the Parmesan cheese and 2 tablespoons (16 g) of the capers. Continue cooking gently for about 2 minutes until the sauce thickens. Stir in the lemon juice and fresh parsley. Taste and adjust the seasonings with salt and pepper if desired.

Add the cooked chicken back into the pan and allow the mixture to simmer until the chicken is coated with sauce and warmed through. Garnish with the remaining 2 tablespoons (16 g) of capers. Serve with roasted potatoes or low-FODMAP, gluten-free capellini.

NUTRITION PER SERVING: Serving Size: 319 g, Calories: 440, Total Fat: 26 g, Saturated Fat: 11 g, Carbohydrates: 7 g, Sugar: 1 g, Sodium: 1340 mg, Fiber: 1 g, Protein: 43 g

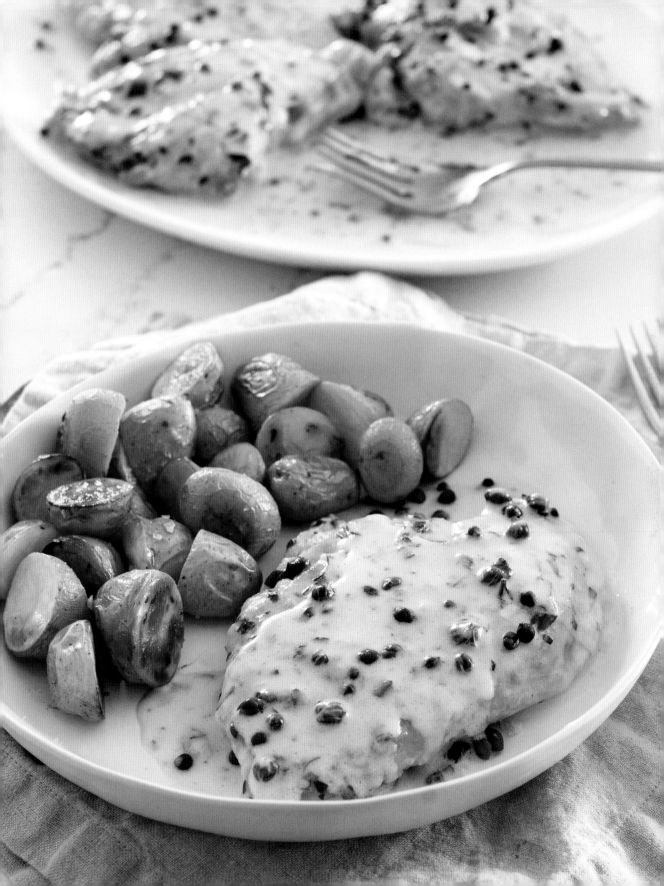

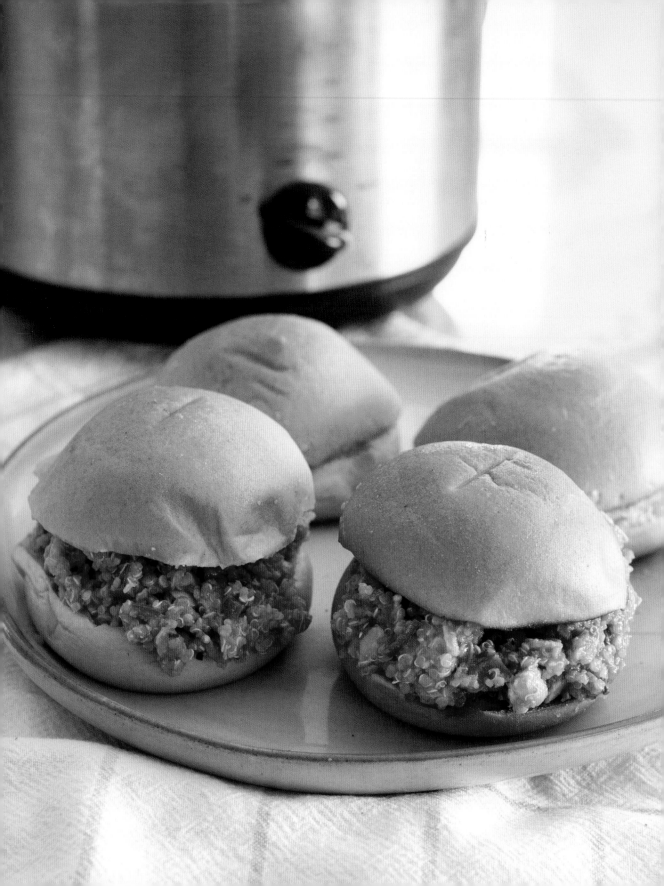

SLOW COOKER VEGAN SLOPPY JOES

I absolutely love my traditional low-FODMAP Sloppy Joe recipe, so I decided to create a version for my vegan friends to enjoy. These vegan Sloppy Joes use a combination of tempeh and quinoa to create the texture and flavor you expect. The best part is you just throw the ingredients in the slow cooker and let it do the work for you.

Using your hands or a grinder, crumble the soy tempeh well. Place all the ingredients, except the buns, in a 5- to 6-quart (4.5 to 5.4 L) slow cooker and stir well to combine. Cover and cook on low for 2 to 3 hours, stirring occasionally. Taste and adjust any seasonings (salt, pepper, sugar). Serve on low-FODMAP, gluten-free buns.

*Make sure there's no added onion or garlic in the tempeh and tomato paste.

TIP: For the best Sloppy Joe experience, brush both sides of the buns with oil and toast on a griddle or skillet over medium-high heat prior to serving.

8 ounces (277 g) plain soy tempeh, gluten-free if necessary*

½ cup (90 g) uncooked quinoa

½ cup (2 ounces [56 g]) diced green bell pepper

2 tablespoons (30 ml) garlic-infused olive oil

1 tablespoon (6 g) chopped scallions, green tips only, or chives

4 ounces (112 g) tomato paste*

3 tablespoons (36 g) light brown sugar, or to taste

1 tablespoon (15 g) yellow mustard

2 teaspoons red wine vinegar

2 teaspoons vegan-certified Worcestershire sauce, gluten-free if necessary

2 cups (470 ml) low-FODMAP vegan broth, gluten-free if necessary (see Note, page 61)

¼ teaspoon salt, plus more to taste

¼ teaspoon pepper, plus more to taste

4 to 6 low-FODMAP buns, for serving, gluten-free if necessary

NUTRITION PER SERVING: Serving Size: 355 g, Calories: 500, Total Fat: 14 g, Saturated Fat: 2 g, Carbohydrates: 77 g, Sugar: 18 g, Sodium: 970 mg, Fiber: 9 g, Protein: 20 g

STIR-FRY GINGER SHRIMP AND VEGETABLES

This is an easy and healthy shrimp stir-fry, tossed in a light sauce of fresh ginger and garlic. Fish sauce is available at most Asian grocery stores and gives this dish extra umami (savory flavor).

1 pound (455 g) uncooked medium shrimp, peeled and deveined, tails on or off

1 tablespoon (15 ml) garlic-infused oil

2 tablespoons (30 ml) low-sodium soy sauce, gluten-free if necessary

1 tablespoon (15 ml) fish sauce

1 tablespoon (15 ml) freshly squeezed lemon juice

1 tablespoon (6 g) grated fresh ginger

¼ teaspoon ground black pepper

1 tablespoon (15 ml) olive oil

3 carrots (200 g), sliced into thin sticks

3 cups (225 g) broccoli florets

1 (8-ounce [227 g]) can bamboo shoots, drained

1 tablespoon (6 g) chopped scallions, green tips only

1 tablespoon (8 g) toasted sesame seeds

Rinse the shrimp and pat dry with a paper towel. In a large bowl, whisk together the infused oil, soy sauce, fish sauce, lemon juice, ginger, and black pepper. Heat the olive oil in a large wok or 12-inch (30 cm) nonstick skillet over medium heat. Add the vegetables to the skillet and stir-fry until the carrots and broccoli are tender-crisp, about 8 minutes. Add the shrimp, then the sauce, and stir-fry until the vegetables are tender and the shrimp is pink and opaque, about 5 minutes. Serve over rice or rice noodles, topped with green scallion tips and sesame seeds.

VARIATION: Add some canned water chestnuts instead of bamboo shoots or use scallops in place of the shrimp.

TIP: Store your fresh ginger in the freezer. It makes it so much easier to grate the amount you need (no need to peel it), and it keeps for months without spoilage.

NUTRITION PER SERVING: Serving Size: 305 g, Calories: 210, Total Fat: 10 g, Saturated Fat: 1.5 g, Carbohydrates: 12 g, Sugar: 5 g, Sodium: 1350 mg, Fiber: 4 g, Protein: 20 g

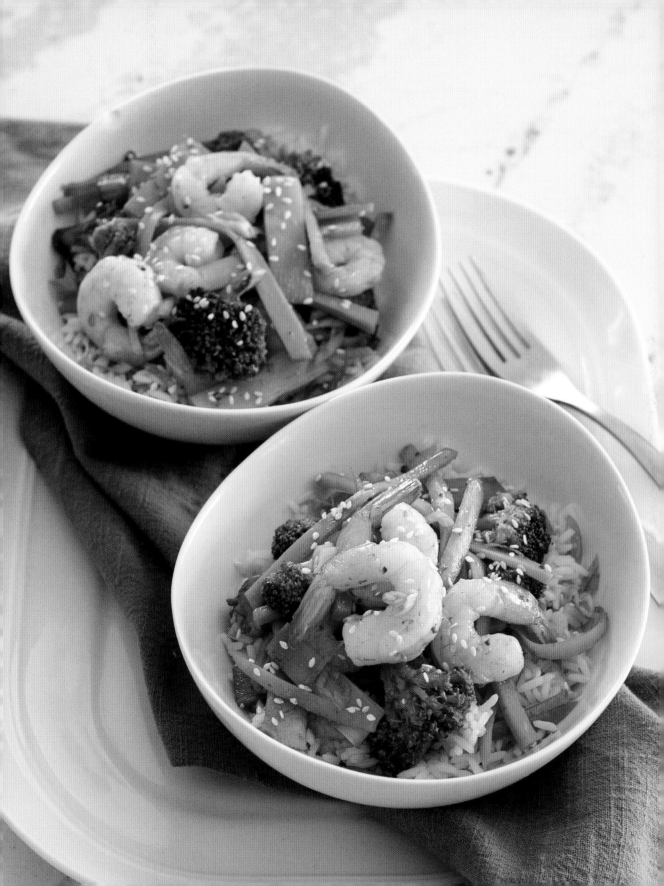

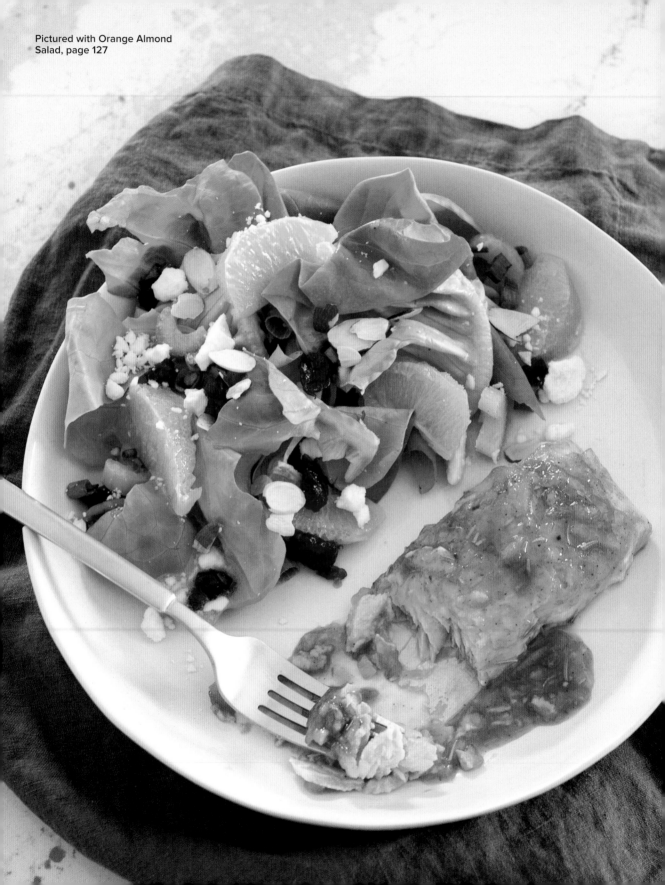

Pictured with Orange Almond
Salad, page 127

ORANGE MARMALADE SALMON

I enjoy salmon at least once a week, and this is my go-to recipe for a quick and tasty meal using ingredients I have on hand. Orange marmalade gives the salmon that sweet and citrusy flavor, while the Dijon provides the perfect contrast. Even if you don't like fish, you will love this recipe.

Preheat the oven to 425°F (220°C, or gas mark 7). Line a large casserole dish or sheet pan with foil and spray with baking spray.

Arrange the salmon fillets in a single layer on the foil, skin-side down. In a small bowl, combine the marmalade, Dijon mustard, maple syrup, infused oil, rosemary, and pepper. Spoon the glaze over the salmon pieces without touching the fish (you don't want to contaminate the glaze with the raw fish). Once they are covered, place the remaining glaze in the refrigerator, and spread the glaze over the entire surface of each fillet. Let the salmon stand for 15 minutes, or place in the fridge for up to 1 hour.

When ready to bake, transfer the salmon to the oven and bake, uncovered, for 15 to 20 minutes, basting occasionally with the pan juices. Salmon is cooked when the surface is glazed and golden and it flakes easily with a fork. Enjoy immediately, or store in the refrigerator; this dish can be served warm or cold. Serve topped with remaining glaze.

NOTE: Salmon is best served slightly rare. Depending on the thickness of your fillets, you may need less time to cook.

6 (6-ounce [170 g]) salmon fillets, skin on or off

¼ cup (80 g) all-natural orange marmalade

¼ cup (60 g) Dijon mustard

2 tablespoons (30 ml) maple syrup

1 teaspoon garlic-infused olive oil

1 teaspoon dried rosemary

½ teaspoon black pepper

NUTRITION PER SERVING: Serving Size: 201 g, Calories: 420, Total Fat: 24 g, Saturated Fat: 5 g, Carbohydrates: 12 g, Sugar: 11 g, Sodium: 340 mg, Fiber: 1 g, Protein: 35 g

SHEET PAN BALSAMIC CHICKEN WITH POTATOES AND VEGETABLES

Savory balsamic and sweet maple combine perfectly in an easy sheet pan chicken and veggie meal. FODMAP fact: Balsamic vinegar is low FODMAP in servings of 1 tablespoon (15 ml).

2 pounds (910 g) baby red and/or gold potatoes, chopped into 1-inch (2.5 cm) slices or small cubes

5 medium carrots (350 g), peeled and chopped into ½-inch (1.3 cm) coins

2 parsnips (100 g), peeled and chopped into ½-inch (1.3 cm) coins

1 pound (455 g, 4 pieces) boneless, skinless chicken breasts, of even thickness

¼ cup (80 g) balsamic vinegar

1 tablespoon (15 g) Dijon mustard

3 tablespoons (45 ml) freshly squeezed lemon juice

⅓ cup (80 ml) maple syrup

2 tablespoons (30 ml) olive oil

1 tablespoon (15 ml) garlic-infused oil

1 teaspoon salt, plus more to taste

½ teaspoon black pepper, plus more to taste

½ teaspoon dried basil

½ teaspoon dried thyme

½ teaspoon dried rosemary

3 tablespoons (18 g) grated Parmesan cheese (omit for dairy-free)

Spray two large rimmed sheet pans with baking spray. Set your oven racks on the upper and lower thirds of the oven and preheat the oven to 400°F (200°C, or gas mark 6).

Arrange the potatoes in a single layer on the first sheet pan, and if there is room, place some of the vegetables on it as well. On the second pan, place your remaining vegetables on one side and the chicken on the other. Be careful not to crowd the vegetables and potatoes; it will slow the cooking.

In a small saucepan, bring the balsamic vinegar, Dijon, lemon juice, and maple syrup to a boil. Cook for about 5 minutes until reduced, then remove from the heat. Drizzle the olive and garlic-infused oil over the potatoes, chicken, carrots, and parsnips. Season everything with salt and pepper, then sprinkle with the basil, thyme, and rosemary. Spoon half of the balsamic sauce over the chicken only. Sprinkle the Parmesan cheese, if using, over the potatoes. Transfer both sheet pans to the oven, with the pan containing the potatoes on the higher rack. Bake for 20 minutes. Flip the chicken and bake for another 10 to 15 minutes until the chicken's internal temperature reaches 165°F (73°C) on a meat thermometer and the vegetables and potatoes are tender (see Note). Drizzle the remaining balsamic sauce over the chicken and vegetables just before serving and season with salt and pepper to taste.

NOTE: Depending how small you cut your vegetables, they may cook slower than the chicken. Once the chicken is cooked, you may remove it to a covered plate and allow the vegetables to continue baking to your desired doneness.

NUTRITION PER SERVING: Serving Size: 533 g, Calories: 550, Total Fat: 15 g, Saturated Fat: 3 g, Carbohydrates: 72 g, Sugar: 28 g, Sodium: 920 mg, Fiber: 8 g, Protein: 32 g

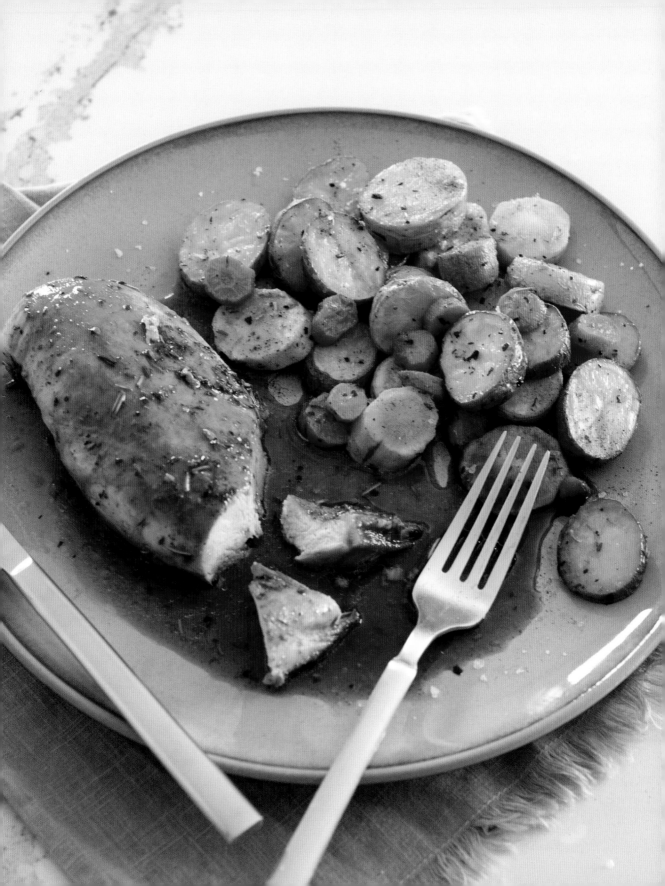

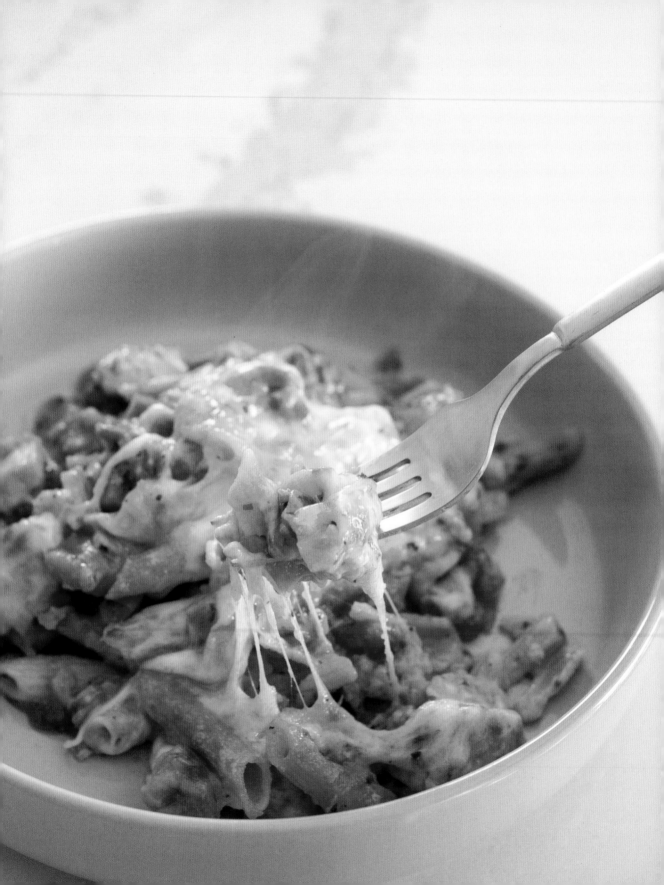

CHEESY CHICKEN PASTA BAKE

You can never go wrong with chicken, cheese, and pasta. This meal was an instant hit at my house. The sauce is rich, herby, and flavorful and tastes gorgeous with the tender chicken thighs and extra cheesy top.

Preheat the oven to 350°F (180°C, or gas mark 4) and place a rack in the center of the oven.

In a large pot, cook the penne pasta according to the package directions until al dente, about 7 minutes, then drain well.

While the pasta is cooking, heat the olive oil in a large oven-safe pan or 6-quart (5.4 L) Dutch oven over medium heat. Add the chicken, green bell pepper, and seasonings and sauté until the chicken is no longer pink, about 10 minutes, adjusting the heat as necessary (the chicken does not need to be cooked through at this point).

In a medium bowl, whisk together the canned tomatoes, tomato paste, chicken broth, and infused oil. Pour the tomato sauce over the chicken and toss to coat. Lower the heat and simmer until the sauce thickens slightly, 10 to 15 minutes. Remove the pan from the heat and add the drained pasta, along with 1 cup (105 g) of the mozzarella and ¼ cup (25 g) of the Parmesan. Stir everything together, then sprinkle the remaining cheeses over the top.

Cover and bake for 20 to 30 minutes, then remove the lid and turn the oven to broil. Return the pan to the oven and bake until the cheese is golden, about 5 more minutes. Serve immediately.

*Select a tomato sauce and paste without added onion and garlic.

VARIATION: You can also use boneless, skinless chicken breasts for this recipe.

TIP: Use kitchen shears to cut your chicken pieces; it's so much easier than using a knife (and safer!).

1½ cups (168 g) uncooked low-FODMAP, gluten-free penne

1 tablespoon (15 ml) olive oil

1½ pounds (680 g) boneless skinless chicken thighs, cut into 1-inch (2.5 cm) pieces

½ cup (75 g) chopped green bell pepper

1 teaspoon dried basil

1 teaspoon dried oregano

1 teaspoon dried parsley flakes

½ teaspoon salt

½ teaspoon black pepper

¼ teaspoon crushed red pepper flakes (optional)

1 (14-ounce [392 g]) can diced tomatoes, undrained*

2 tablespoons (30 g) tomato paste*

1 cup (235 ml) low-FODMAP chicken broth, gluten-free if necessary (see Note, page 61)

1 tablespoon (15 ml) garlic-infused oil

2 cups (210 g) shredded mozzarella cheese, divided

½ cup (50 g) grated fresh Parmesan, divided

NUTRITION PER SERVING: Serving Size: 315 g, Calories: 430, Total Fat: 18 g, Saturated Fat: 7 g, Carbohydrates: 29 g, Sugar: 3 g, Sodium: 920 mg, Fiber: 2 g, Protein: 37 g

Yield: 12 servings   **Prep time:** 20 minutes   **Bake time:** 50 to 60 minutes

"KEY LIME" LOAF

While Key limes have not been formally tested for FODMAP content, you can enjoy a similar flavor by using a combination of fresh lemon and lime juice and zest. This lemon-lime loaf is soft and light, with a tantalizing tartness from the creamy glaze.

FOR THE KEY LIME LOAF:

Vegetable shortening, for greasing

2 cups (240 g) low-FODMAP, gluten-free flour

2 teaspoons baking powder

½ teaspoon salt

¾ teaspoon xanthan gum*

1 cup (200 g) granulated sugar

3 large eggs, at room temperature

¾ cup (180 ml) low-FODMAP milk, such as lactose-free or almond milk

2 teaspoons grated lemon zest

1 teaspoon grated lime zest

3 tablespoons (45 ml) freshly squeezed lemon juice (about 1 medium lemon)

1 tablespoon (15 ml) freshly squeezed lime juice (about ½ medium lime)

½ cup (120 ml) canola or avocado oil

½ teaspoon Key lime extract**

FOR THE KEY LIME GLAZE:

2 tablespoons (30 ml) freshly squeezed lemon juice

1 tablespoon (15 ml) freshly squeezed lime juice

1½ cups (180 g) confectioners' sugar

1 to 2 tablespoons (15 to 30 ml) low-FODMAP milk, such as lactose-free or almond milk, as needed

Lime zest, for garnish

To make the loaf: Preheat the oven to 350°F (180°C, or gas mark 4) and place a rack in the center of the oven. Grease a 9 x 5-inch (23 x 13 cm) loaf pan with shortening and line with parchment paper with a 1-inch (2.5 cm) overhang. Grease the parchment paper with shortening as well.

In a large bowl, combine the flour, baking powder, salt, xanthan gum (if needed), and granulated sugar.

Beat the eggs in a separate large bowl with a hand mixer, or use a stand mixer with the paddle attachment. Add the low-FODMAP milk, lemon zest, and lime zest to the eggs, then slowly add the lemon and lime juices, followed by the oil and Key lime extract. Add the dry ingredients to the wet ingredients and mix on low until just combined. Transfer the batter to the prepared loaf pan. Bake for 50 to 60 minutes until a tester inserted into the center of the loaf comes out clean and the top is slightly spongy to the touch. Let the loaf sit in the pan for about 10 minutes, then use the overhanging parchment paper to remove it from the pan and transfer to a rack to cool completely.

To make the glaze: Combine the lemon and lime juices in a medium bowl. Gradually add the confectioners' sugar and whisk until smooth and creamy. Add the milk, 1 teaspoon at a time, to thin as needed. When the loaf has cooled to room temperature, evenly spread the glaze over the top of the loaf and sprinkle with the lime zest. Serve immediately, or store in an airtight container at room temperature.

*Only add xanthan gum if it is not already listed as an ingredient in your low-FODMAP flour.

**If you can't find Key lime extract, then use lime or lemon extract instead. It will taste slightly different but will still be delicious.

TIP: Select a high-quality finely ground rice flour blend for the best rise and texture. I like Authentic Foods GF Classical Blend for my baking. Corn flours, while gluten-free, do not make the best baked goods.

NUTRITION PER SERVING: Serving Size: 81 g, Calories: 250, Total Fat: 11 g, Saturated Fat: 1.5 g, Carbohydrates: 35 g, Sugar: 18 g, Sodium: 210 mg, Fiber: 1 g, Protein: 3 g

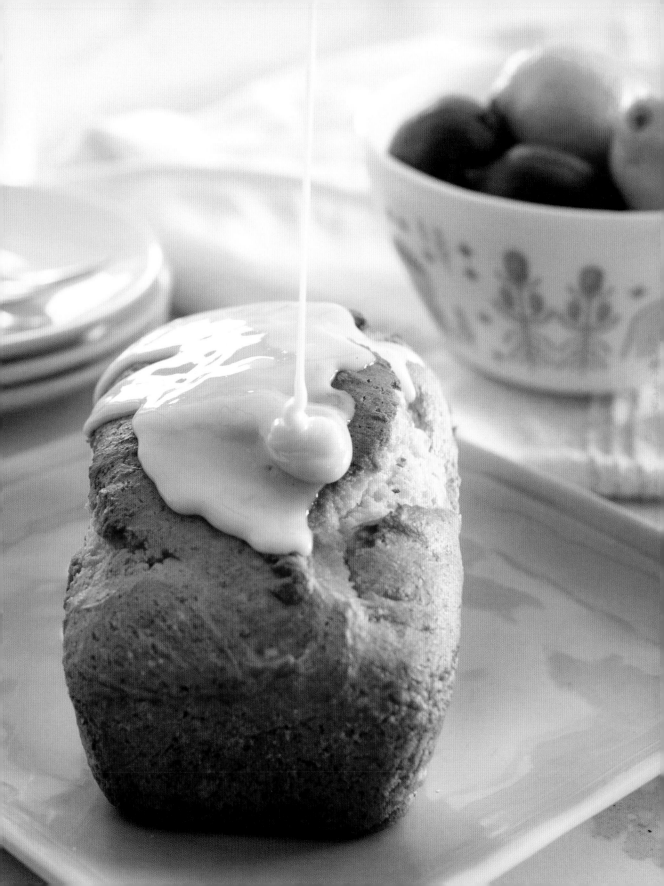

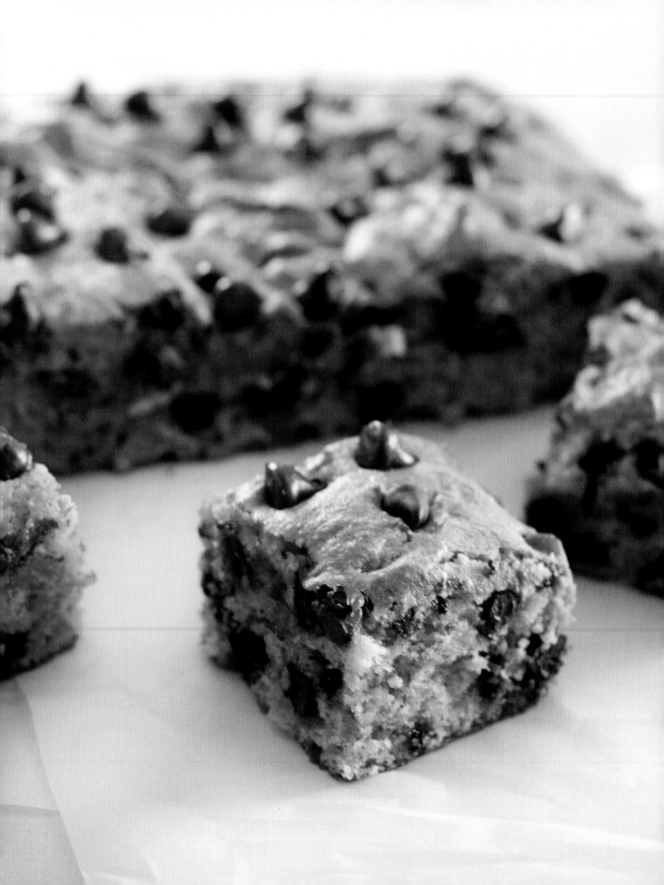

BANANA BLONDIES WITH CHOCOLATE CHIPS

I prefer blondies over brownies, but banana blondies may be the best of all. The banana adds extra flavor and moisture while creating the perfect fudgy texture. Of course, you can't skip the chocolate chips, especially in my household!

Preheat the oven to 350°F (180°C, or gas mark 4) and place a rack in the center of the oven. Line an 8-inch (20 cm) square baking pan with parchment paper or aluminum foil with a 1- to 2-inch (2.5 to 5 cm) overhang. Spray the paper or foil with baking spray or grease with shortening.

In a large bowl, combine the almond meal, flour, xanthan gum (if needed), baking powder, cinnamon, and salt.

In a separate large bowl, use a hand mixer or a stand mixer fitted with the paddle attachment to cream the butter and light brown sugar together. Add the eggs, mashed banana, and vanilla to the butter mixture, and mix well on medium-low. Add the dry ingredients to the wet ingredients and mix on low until just combined. Stir in the chocolate chips by hand. Spread the batter evenly into the prepared pan. Top with a few extra chips for decoration if desired.

Bake for 25 to 35 minutes, or until a toothpick inserted into the center comes out clean. Let cool in the pan for 45 minutes or longer. Slice into 16 bars to serve. Store leftovers in an airtight container at room temperature.

*Only add xanthan gum if it is not already listed as an ingredient in your low-FODMAP flour.

NOTE: Bananas get sweeter as they ripen because the carbohydrates in them convert from starch to sugar. This means a riper banana is higher in FODMAP content. For a ripe banana, about ⅓ of the banana, or 35 g, makes up one low-FODMAP serving (see "FODMAP FAQs," page 20, for other details).

¾ cup (90 g) almond meal or almond flour

¾ cup (90 g) low-FODMAP, gluten-free flour

½ teaspoon xanthan gum*

1 teaspoon baking powder

1 teaspoon ground cinnamon

¼ teaspoon salt

⅓ cup (75 g) butter or low-FODMAP, dairy-free butter alternative, softened

¾ cup (150 g) light brown sugar, packed

2 large eggs, at room temperature

⅔ cup (170 g) mashed ripe banana

1 teaspoon vanilla extract

1 cup (170 g) semisweet chocolate chips (dairy-free if necessary), plus a few for sprinkling

NUTRITION PER SERVING: Serving Size: 54 g, Calories: 190, Total Fat: 10 g, Saturated Fat: 4.5 g, Carbohydrates: 26 g, Sugar: 17 g, Sodium: 110 mg, Fiber: 2 g, Protein: 3 g

SHOW-STOPPING LEMON OLIVE OIL CAKE

Olive oil cakes are a traditional Italian dessert. The ideal version should be moist and rich, with an almost pudding-like interior. My olive oil cake is infused with fresh lemon flavor and has added texture from almond meal. A showstopper at any occasion.

FOR THE CAKE:

1 cup (235 ml) good-quality olive oil (see Tip), plus more for greasing and brushing the cake

2 cups (400 g) granulated sugar, plus more for sprinkling in the pan

1½ cups (180 g) low-FODMAP, gluten-free flour

¼ cup (30 g) tapioca starch or flour

¼ cup (30 g) almond meal

¾ teaspoon xanthan gum*

½ teaspoon baking soda

½ teaspoon baking powder

1 teaspoon salt

1½ cups (355 ml) low-FODMAP milk, such as lactose-free or almond milk

½ cup (120 ml) freshly squeezed lemon juice (2 to 3 medium lemons)

1 tablespoon (6 g) finely grated lemon zest (about 1 medium lemon)

2 teaspoons vanilla extract

3 large eggs, at room temperature

Confectioners' sugar, for dusting (if not using glaze)

To make the cake: Preheat the oven to 350°F (180°C, or gas mark 4) and place a rack in the center of the oven. Use wax paper or your hand to coat the sides of a 9-inch (23 cm) round springform cake pan with olive oil. Cut a piece of parchment paper into a circle and place in the bottom of the pan and grease this as well. Wrap the base of the pan in aluminum foil to seal the edges. Sprinkle granulated sugar over the pan bottom and set aside.

In a medium bowl, combine the flour, tapioca starch, almond meal, xanthan gum (if needed), baking soda, baking powder, and salt.

In a second medium bowl, add the milk, then stir in the lemon juice, lemon zest, and vanilla. Don't worry if the milk curdles; this is a normal reaction when you add an acid like lemon.

In a third large bowl, cream together the eggs and granulated sugar using a hand mixer, or use a stand mixer fitted with the paddle attachment. Beat on high until well incorporated, pale, and thick, about 3 minutes. Drizzle in the olive oil slowly and beat until completely combined (it will be quite yellow). Add the dry ingredients in four stages, alternating with the lemon juice mixture, while the mixer is on low. You should finish with the dry ingredients. Scrape down the sides and bottom of the bowl as needed and be careful not to overmix.

Pour the batter into your prepared cake pan and place in the center of the oven. Bake for 80 to 90 minutes, or until the cake springs back to the touch and a tester inserted in the middle comes out clean or with only scant moist crumbs (since ovens vary, your oven may need more or less time).

Continued on page 94

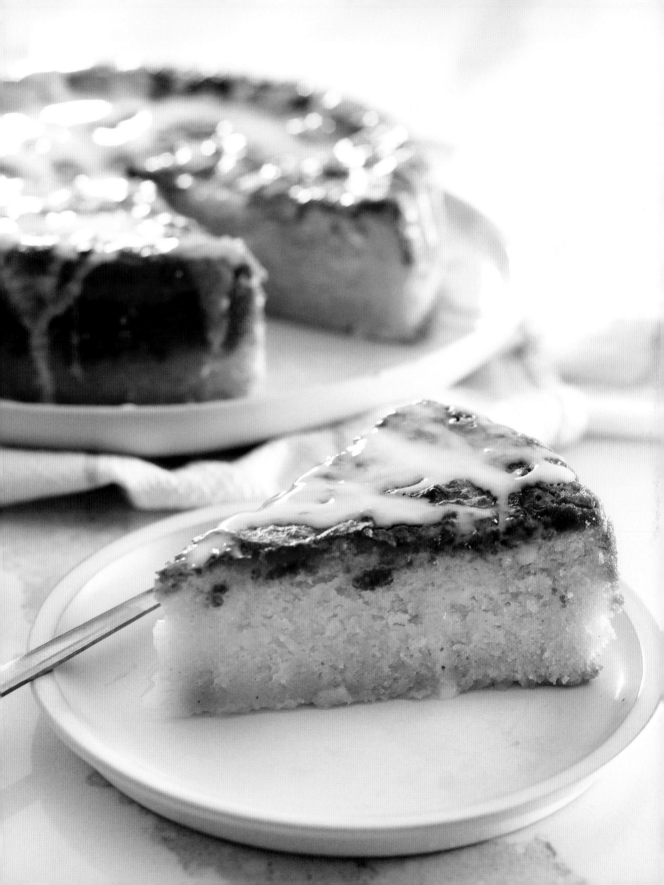

continued from page 92

FOR THE LEMON GLAZE (OPTIONAL):

1 cup (120 g) confectioners' sugar

2 to 3 tablespoons (30 to 45 ml) lemon juice

Remove the cake from the oven and let cool for 10 minutes in the pan on a rack. Then use a knife to separate the cake from the sides of the pan and release the spring to remove the sides. Leave the cake pan bottom attached and allow the cake to cool on the rack until it is room temperature. Carefully remove the parchment paper from the cake and transfer to a cake platter.

To make the glaze: Mix the confectioners' sugar with the lemon juice a little at a time until you've reached your desired consistency.

Brush the cooled cake with additional olive oil and sprinkle with confectioners' sugar, or drizzle with the lemon glaze. Cover the cake with plastic wrap or a lid, and store at room temperature until serving.

*Only add xanthan gum if it is not already listed as an ingredient in your low-FODMAP flour.

TIP: For a cake like this, the quality of the oil will make a big difference. Skip your regular cooking oil for a finer quality extra-virgin olive oil with an aromatic flavor profile. Basically, if you wouldn't use it on a salad, then don't bake this cake with it.

NUTRITION PER SERVING: Serving Size: 95 g, Calories: 300, Total Fat: 16 g, Saturated Fat: 2.5 g, Carbohydrates: 38 g, Sugar: 26 g, Sodium: 230 mg, Fiber: 1 g, Protein: 3 g

"OATSTANDING" OATMEAL, CHOCOLATE, AND PEANUT BUTTER COOKIES

My chewy oatmeal no-bake cookies are easy, tasty, and healthy—an "oatstanding" choice for snacking. Packed with protein and fiber, they will give you energy for a long afternoon or after a workout. Prepare these in just 15 minutes and have a lovely treat all week long.

Line two large rimmed baking sheets with parchment paper or silicone baking mats.

Place the butter, sugar, milk, cocoa powder, and salt in a large saucepan over medium heat. Bring the mixture to a boil and let boil for 1 minute. Remove the pan from the heat, then add the peanut butter, vanilla, and cinnamon (if using). Stir until smooth, then add the oats a little at a time until combined. Scoop the dough onto the prepared sheets using a medium cookie scoop and slightly flatten the tops. Chill in the refrigerator or at room temperature until set. Cookies may be stored at room temperature or in the refrigerator for up to 2 weeks.

NOTE: A no-stir peanut butter will give you the best results here. If your brand is on the thick side, then you can add some peanut or canola oil to smooth out the batter.

½ cup (112 g) unsalted butter

2 cups (400 g) sugar

½ cup (120 ml) low-FODMAP milk, such as lactose-free or almond milk

¼ cup (32 g) unsweetened cocoa powder

¼ teaspoon salt

½ cup (120 g) all-natural, no-stir peanut butter (see Note)

2 teaspoons vanilla extract

1 teaspoon ground cinnamon (optional)

3 cups (240 g) traditional (old-fashioned) rolled oats

NUTRITION PER SERVING: Serving Size: 43 g, Calories: 170, Total Fat: 7 g, Saturated Fat: 3 g, Carbohydrates: 25 g, Sugar: 18 g, Sodium: 50 mg, Fiber: 2 g, Protein: 3 g

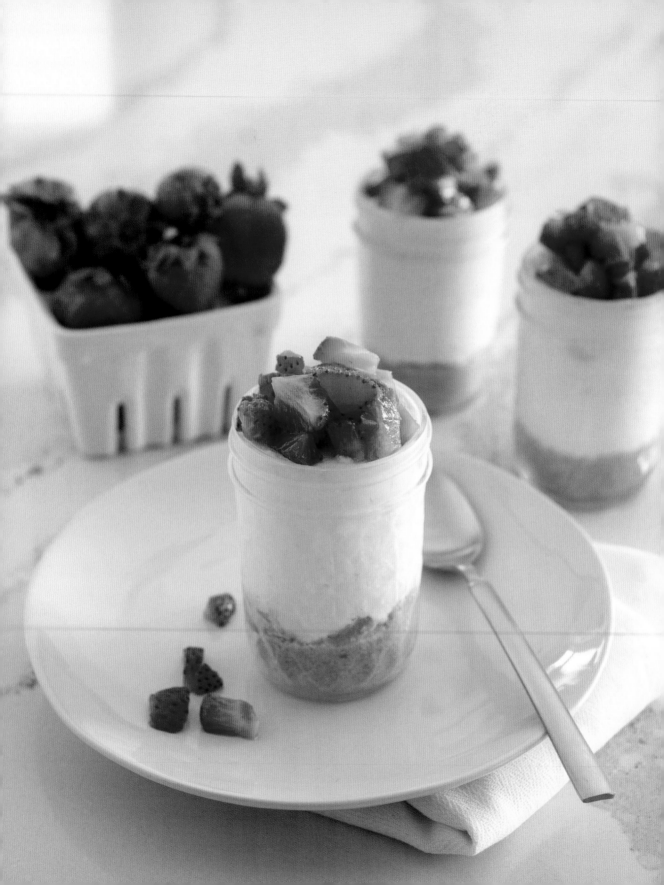

NO-BAKE STRAWBERRY CHEESECAKE JARS

No-bake cheesecake jars are the sweetest treat to have at a brunch, summer barbecue, or bridal shower. They look so pretty served in individual tulip jars or mason jars. I decorate mine with fresh flowers and pink sprinkles. FODMAP fact: Strawberries are low FODMAP in servings of 65 g.

Wash and dry six 8-ounce (227 g) mason or tulip jars (you can also use glasses) and set aside.

Process the cookies in your food processor until they're reduced to a fine crumb. Add the melted butter a bit at a time and pulse until the mixture is well combined and clumps together (depending on which cookies you're using, you may need more or less butter). Evenly divide the cookies among the six jars, pressing the crumbs into the bottom of your jars to create a flat base. Place the jars in the refrigerator to chill.

Slice the strawberries and add them to a resealable bag with ½ teaspoon of the lemon juice and 1 tablespoon (12 g) of the sugar. Place the bag in the fridge as well to chill.

Beat the whipping cream in a medium bowl using an electric mixer until stiff peaks form, about 3 minutes. In a separate bowl, beat the cream cheese, sour cream, remaining ⅓ cup (65 g) of sugar, remaining 1 teaspoon of lemon juice, and vanilla until smooth and creamy, about 1 minute. Gently fold the whipped cream into this mixture by hand.

Remove the jars from the fridge and add the cheesecake mixture to them, evenly distributing it among the jars. Return the jars to the fridge to chill for at least 30 minutes. Top with the strawberry mixture before serving. Cheesecakes may be stored in the refrigerator for up to 5 days.

VARIATION: I like a thick cookie crust on the bottom, but if you prefer less, then use 100 g of cookies and 2 to 3 teaspoons of coconut oil instead.

TIP: For this recipe I like to use gluten-free white sandwich cookies, such as Glutino or Goodie Girl brands, or shortbread cookies such as Walkers brand. Whichever cookie you choose, check that your product contains low-FODMAP ingredients or is FODMAP tested.

NOTE: Lactose-free cream cheese tends to be watery. I strain mine well before use to reduce this.

8 ounces (200 g) low-FODMAP, gluten-free cookies of your choice (see Tip)

1 to 2 tablespoons (15 to 30 g) unsalted butter or coconut oil, melted

1¼ cups (260 g) fresh strawberries, hulled

1½ teaspoons freshly squeezed lemon juice, divided

⅓ cup plus 1 tablespoon (78 g) granulated sugar, divided

1 cup (235 ml) heavy whipping cream, chilled

8 ounces (227 g) lactose-free cream cheese, strained

2 tablespoons (30 g) lactose-free or regular full-fat sour cream

½ teaspoon vanilla extract

NUTRITION PER SERVING: Serving Size: 176 g, Calories: 540, Total Fat: 39 g, Saturated Fat: 24 g, Carbohydrates: 46 g, Sugar: 33 g, Sodium: 180 mg, Fiber: 1 g, Protein: 4 g

CINNAMON STREUSEL ZUCCHINI COFFEE CAKE

For those of you who are unfamiliar with the term, "coffee cake" is not a coffee-*flavored* cake but rather a cake that you enjoy *with your coffee*. This low-FODMAP version gets moisture and nutritional benefits from zucchini, and gorgeous flavor from the spices and streusel topping.

FOR THE STREUSEL TOPPING:

¾ cup (90 g) low-FODMAP, gluten-free flour

¼ cup (50 g) granulated sugar

¼ cup (60 g) packed light brown sugar

¼ teaspoon salt

1 teaspoon ground cinnamon

6 tablespoons (90 g) unsalted butter or coconut oil, melted

½ cup (75 g) chopped pecans or walnuts

FOR THE COFFEE CAKE:

2 large eggs, at room temperature

1 cup (200 g) granulated sugar

About 1¼ cups (226 g) packed finely grated zucchini, patted dry (see Tip)

½ cup (120 ml) canola or avocado oil

2 teaspoons ground cinnamon

2 teaspoons vanilla extract

1 cup (120 g) low-FODMAP, gluten-free flour

¼ teaspoon xanthan gum*

1 teaspoon baking powder

½ teaspoon baking soda

¼ teaspoon salt

FOR THE VANILLA GLAZE:

¾ cup (90 g) confectioners' sugar

1 tablespoon (15 ml) low-FODMAP milk, such as lactose-free or almond milk

½ teaspoon vanilla extract

Preheat the oven to 350°F (180°C, or gas mark 4) and place a rack in the center of the oven. Line an 8-inch (20 cm) square pan with aluminum foil or parchment paper (optional) and spray with baking spray; set aside.

To make the streusel topping: Place the flour, both sugars, salt, and cinnamon in a medium bowl and stir to combine. Drizzle in the melted butter. Stir and "fluff" the mixture with your fork; it should be crumbly and clumpy. Add the chopped pecans and lightly mix again. Set aside.

To make the cake: In a large bowl, place the eggs, granulated sugar, zucchini, oil, cinnamon, and vanilla and whisk to combine. In a second large bowl, stir together the flour, xanthan gum (if needed), baking powder, baking soda, and salt. Slowly add the flour mixture to the zucchini mixture and mix by hand until well combined. Spread the batter into the prepared pan, smoothing the top with your spatula. Sprinkle the streusel topping evenly over the cake batter (there is a lot of streusel; I don't skimp on it!). Transfer the pan to the oven and bake for about 50 minutes or until the center is set and a toothpick inserted in the middle comes out clean or with a few moist crumbs. Set the cake in the pan on a wire rack to cool before serving.

To make the glaze: While the cake is cooling, in a bowl, combine the confectioners' sugar with the milk, a little at a time, until you've reached your desired consistency. Stir in the vanilla. When the cake is cool, drizzle the glaze over the top. Store at room temperature in a covered container for up to 5 days.

*Only add xanthan gum if it is not already listed as an ingredient in your low-FODMAP flour.

TIP: I strongly recommend using a scale to ensure you get the correct amount of zucchini for this recipe.

NUTRITION PER SERVING: Serving Size: 80 g, Calories: 300, Total Fat: 16 g, Saturated Fat: 4 g, Carbohydrates: 39 g, Sugar: 26 g, Sodium: 160 mg, Fiber: 1 g, Protein: 2 g

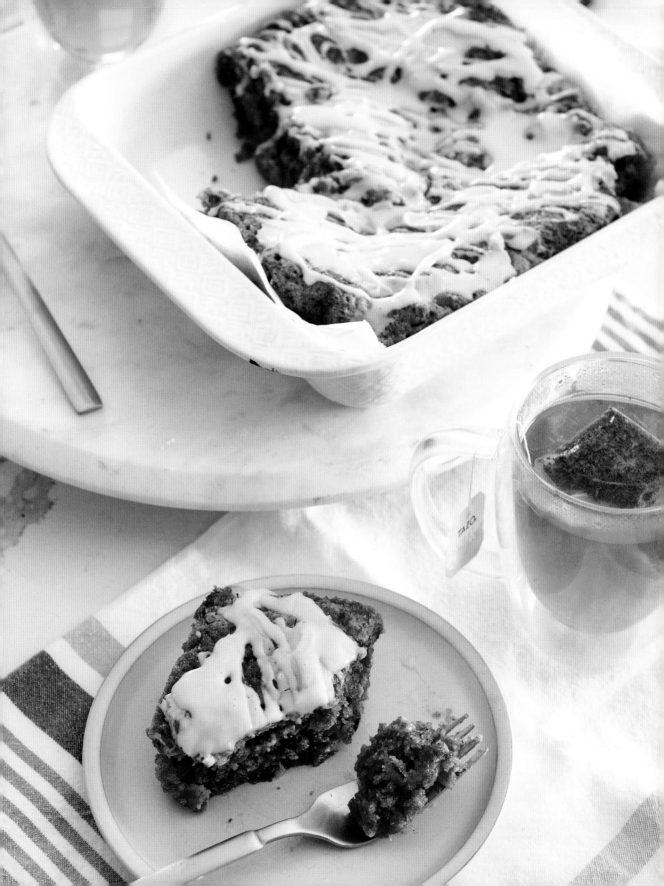

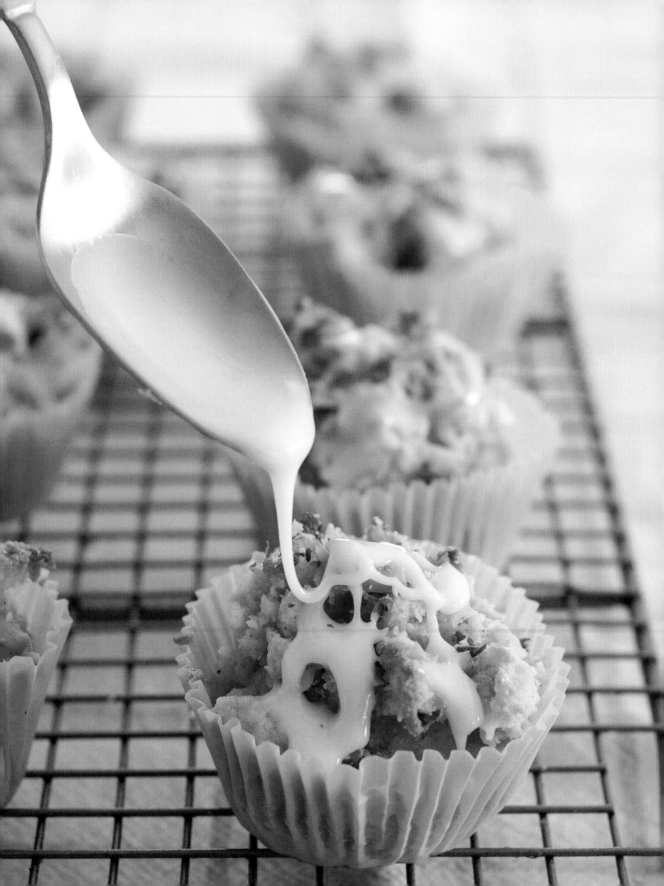

GLAZED PINEAPPLE WALNUT MUFFINS

Moist, sweet, and oh-so-delicious, these muffins are delightful on any summer table. Pineapple is one of my favorite fruits on the low-FODMAP diet; canned pineapple makes this recipe a snap.

To make the muffins: Preheat the oven to 350°F (180°C, or gas mark 4) and place a rack in the center of the oven. Grease a 12-well muffin tin with vegetable shortening or spray with baking spray and line with muffin cups, if desired.

Place the pineapple in a strainer over a medium bowl and press it well with your hands to drain the juice. Reserve the juice in the bowl to use for your glaze. Remove the pineapple from the strainer and pat it dry with a paper towel. Use a scale to weigh your pineapple after draining to make sure you have the correct amount.

Combine the flour, granulated sugar, baking powder, baking soda, xanthan gum (if needed), salt, and cinnamon in a large bowl. Stir in ½ cup (75 g) of the walnuts, reserving the rest for sprinkling.

In a second medium bowl, whisk together the milk and oil. Remove 1 tablespoon (15 ml) of the combined liquid and discard it. Add the eggs and vanilla to the bowl and beat well to combine, then stir in the pineapple. Add the wet ingredients to the dry ingredients and mix well by hand. Using a large cookie scoop, fill the muffin wells evenly, about three-fourths full, and sprinkle the remaining walnuts on top. Transfer the muffins to the oven and bake for 22 to 28 minutes, until the tops are golden brown and a tester inserted into the center of a muffin comes out clean. Let the muffins cool in the pan on a wire rack for 3 to 5 minutes, then remove from the pan to cool completely on the rack.

To make the glaze: Mix the confectioners' sugar and reserved pineapple juice in a medium bowl to your desired consistency. When the muffins are completely cool, drizzle the glaze over the top. Store in an airtight container at room temperature.

*Only add xanthan gum if it is not already listed as an ingredient in your low-FODMAP flour.

VARIATION: You can substitute chocolate chips, white chocolate chips, or fresh blueberries for the walnuts if you prefer.

NOTE: Canned pineapple "in syrup" has higher amounts of FODMAPs; do not substitute.

FOR THE MUFFINS:

1 cup (226 g) canned crushed pineapple "in juice" (see Note)

2 cups (240 g) low-FODMAP, gluten-free flour

1 cup (200 g) granulated sugar

1 tablespoon (8 g) baking powder

1 teaspoon baking soda

¾ teaspoon xanthan gum*

¼ teaspoon salt

½ teaspoon ground cinnamon

¾ cup (100 g) chopped walnuts, divided

½ cup (120 ml) low-FODMAP milk, such as lactose-free or almond milk

½ cup (120 ml) canola or avocado oil

2 large eggs, at room temperature

1 teaspoon vanilla extract

FOR THE PINEAPPLE GLAZE:

¾ cup (90 g) confectioners' sugar

1 to 2 tablespoons (15 to 30 ml) reserved pineapple juice

NUTRITION PER SERVING: Serving Size: 101 g, Calories: 330, Total Fat: 16 g, Saturated Fat: 1.5 g, Carbohydrates: 46 g, Sugar: 28 g, Sodium: 250 mg, Fiber: 1 g, Protein: 4 g

DECADENT CHOCOLATE RASPBERRY MUG CAKE

Decadent simplicity at its best. A personal-sized chocolate mug cake that is ready in about 5 minutes, with raspberries for extra flavor. This is a fabulous snack when you don't want to get out your mixing bowls or turn on a hot oven.

1 egg

¼ cup (30 g) low-FODMAP, gluten-free flour

¼ cup (50 g) granulated sugar

1 tablespoon (8 g) unsweetened cocoa powder

⅛ teaspoon xanthan gum*

⅛ teaspoon baking powder

Pinch of salt

3 tablespoons (45 ml) low-FODMAP milk, such as lactose-free or almond milk

3 tablespoons (45 ml) canola or avocado oil

¼ teaspoon vanilla extract

1 tablespoon (10 g) semisweet chocolate chips, dairy-free if necessary

5 to 6 (25 g) raspberries

Confectioners' sugar, for dusting

Crack the egg into a small bowl, give it a good whisk, then measure out 2 tablespoons (30 ml) into a 10-ounce (280 ml) microwave-safe mug. Add the flour, granulated sugar, cocoa powder, xanthan gum (if needed), baking powder, salt, milk, oil, and vanilla to the mug and whisk to combine. Stuff one or two chocolate chips into the center of the raspberries and fold the raspberries into the batter so they are below the surface. Sprinkle extra chocolate chips on top. Microwave the mug cake on high for 1½ to 2 minutes, watching closely so it doesn't bubble over. The cake should puff up to the rim, then recede back as it cools. Remove the cake from the microwave, and let it stand for about a minute to continue cooking. Sprinkle with the confectioners' sugar before serving.

*Only add xanthan gum if it is not already listed as an ingredient in your low-FODMAP flour.

VARIATION: Try this mug cake with white chocolate chips, instead of semisweet, or pecans or toasted walnuts instead of raspberries.

NUTRITION PER SERVING: Serving Size: 132 g, Calories: 420, Total Fat: 26 g, Saturated Fat: 3.5 g, Carbohydrates: 46 g, Sugar: 30 g, Sodium: 130 mg, Fiber: 3 g, Protein: 6 g

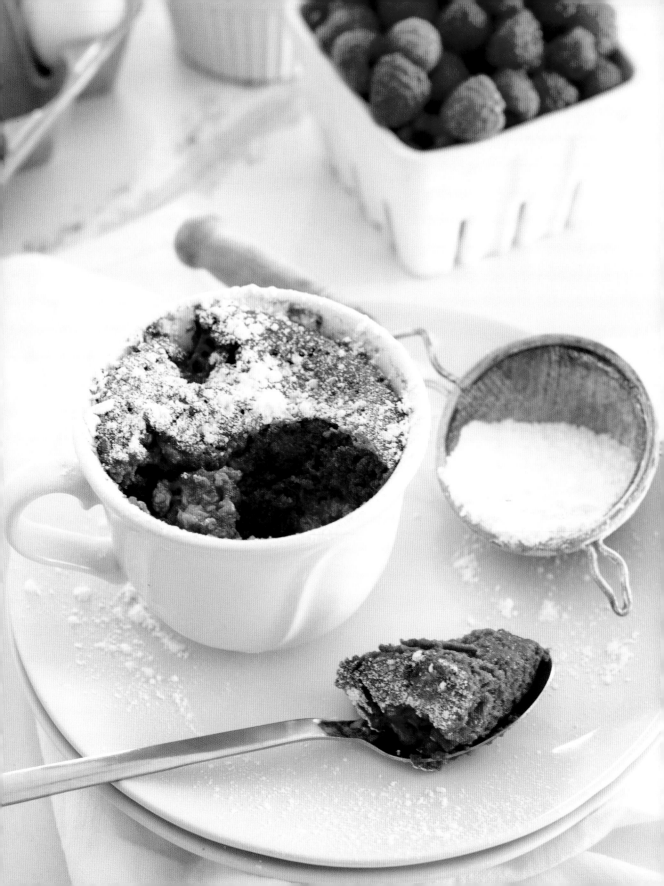

IRRESISTIBLE PUMPKIN-SPICED GRANOLA

I declare my homemade granola to be the *best ever*, and this version uses all my favorite elements: coconut flakes, pepitas, pecans, and the warm flavors of pumpkin pie spices. Let a bowl sit overnight in the fridge with some low-FODMAP milk and you will wake up to amazing granola-flavored overnight oats.

3 cups (240 g) traditional (old-fashioned) rolled oats

2 teaspoons pumpkin pie spice

½ teaspoon salt

1 cup (65 g) unsweetened coconut flakes (not shredded coconut)

¼ cup (25 g) pumpkin seeds or pepitas

¾ cup (70 g) pecan halves

¼ cup (60 ml) melted coconut oil

¼ cup (50 g) brown sugar

¼ cup (65 g) canned pure pumpkin

½ teaspoon vanilla extract

½ cup (120 ml) maple syrup

½ cup (85 g) semisweet vegan chocolate chips (optional) or dried cranberries

Preheat the oven to 300°F (150°C, or gas mark 2) and line a large rimmed baking sheet with aluminum foil or a silicone baking mat.

Combine the oats, pumpkin pie spice, salt, coconut flakes, pumpkin seeds, and pecans in a large bowl. In a second medium bowl, stir together the melted coconut oil, brown sugar, pumpkin, vanilla, and maple syrup. Add the wet ingredients to the oats mixture and stir to combine.

Spread the oat mixture flat on the baking sheet and transfer to the oven. Bake for 20 to 25 minutes. Stir the oats with a spatula and then return to the oven to finish baking for another 20 minutes. If you prefer your oats to be extra crispy, then turn the oven up to 350°F (180°C, or gas mark 4) and bake for a further 5 to 10 minutes.

When the oats are done, remove the sheet from the oven and let cool to room temperature. Stir in the chocolate chips or dried cranberries, if desired. Store in a sealed container or freeze if desired.

TIPS:

+ Try this granola over yogurt or ice cream, or enjoy it plain. It's a super crunchy, satisfying snack.

+ You can freeze leftover canned pumpkin for later! Save it to use in the Mini Pumpkin Biscuits with Cream Cheese Frosting (page 36).

NUTRITION PER SERVING: Serving Size: 41 g, Calories: 180, Total Fat: 10 g, Saturated Fat: 5 g, Carbohydrates: 20 g, Sugar: 9 g, Sodium: 65 mg, Fiber: 2 g, Protein: 3 g

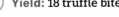
BROWNIE TRUFFLE BITES

No one can resist a bite-sized brownie truffle. These little balls explode with chocolate flavor and are ready in less than 30 minutes. Because raw flour has been associated with bacterial contamination, I will teach you how to "heat treat" your flour in the microwave or oven. It's easy!

Line a large baking sheet with parchment paper or a silicone liner.

Begin by heat treating your flour. To microwave, place your flour in a microwave-safe bowl and heat on high for 50 to 60 seconds. If you prefer to bake, preheat the oven to 350°F (180°C, or gas mark 4) and place a rack in the center of the oven. Spread the flour on a large baking sheet and bake for approximately 10 minutes. With either method, ensure that the internal temperature of the flour reaches 166°F (75°C); increase the cook time as needed. Once it reaches the proper temperature, place the flour in a medium bowl to cool.

In a large bowl with an electric mixer or in a stand mixer, cream the butter and sugar together on high until the sugar granules are mostly dissolved, about 3 minutes. Add the vanilla and beat until creamy, another 2 minutes, scraping the bowl as needed.

Add the cocoa, salt, and espresso powder to the cooled flour and mix well to remove any lumps. Place the flour mixture in the bowl with the creamed butter and beat on low until smooth, about 2 minutes, scraping the bowl as necessary. With a wooden spoon, stir in the chocolate chips.

Using a small cookie scoop, scoop out bite-sized balls of dough and roll them between your palms. (If you prefer the balls even smaller, use a spoon or melon baller to scoop the dough.) Roll the finished balls in cocoa powder or confectioner's sugar, if desired, then place them on the prepared baking sheet. Serve bites immediately, or store them in a covered container at room temperature or in the refrigerator for 3 to 4 days.

TIPS:

+ If your dough is dry when rolling the balls, add 1 teaspoon of low-FODMAP milk or cream until the desired consistency is reached.

+ Caster sugar is a finely ground sugar that results in a smooth texture for these brownie bites. If you don't have it, you can make your own! Simply pulse granulated white sugar in a food processor until it reaches a finely ground, but not powdered, consistency.

¾ cup (120 g) low-FODMAP, gluten-free flour

½ cup (113 g) unsalted butter, room temperature, or low-FODMAP vegan spread

¾ cup (150 g) caster sugar (see Tip)

1 teaspoon vanilla extract

⅓ cup (35 g) cocoa powder

½ teaspoon table salt

½ teaspoon espresso powder (see Note)

½ cup (90 g) mini semisweet vegan chocolate chips

Cocoa powder or confectioner's sugar, optional, for rolling

NOTE: Espresso powder is not the same as instant coffee or instant espresso grinds. It is a very fine powder made from espresso beans that have been brewed and dried. A little goes a long way in enhancing the depth and flavor of chocolate desserts, without tasting "like coffee." You can find espresso powder in the baking aisle of most gourmet grocery stores (or on Amazon). I like King Arthur brand.

NUTRITION PER SERVING: Serving Size: 29 g, Calories: 130, Total Fat: 7 g, Saturated Fat: 4 g, Carbohydrates: 18 g, Sugar: 11 g, Sodium: 70 mg, Fiber: 1 g, Protein: 1 g

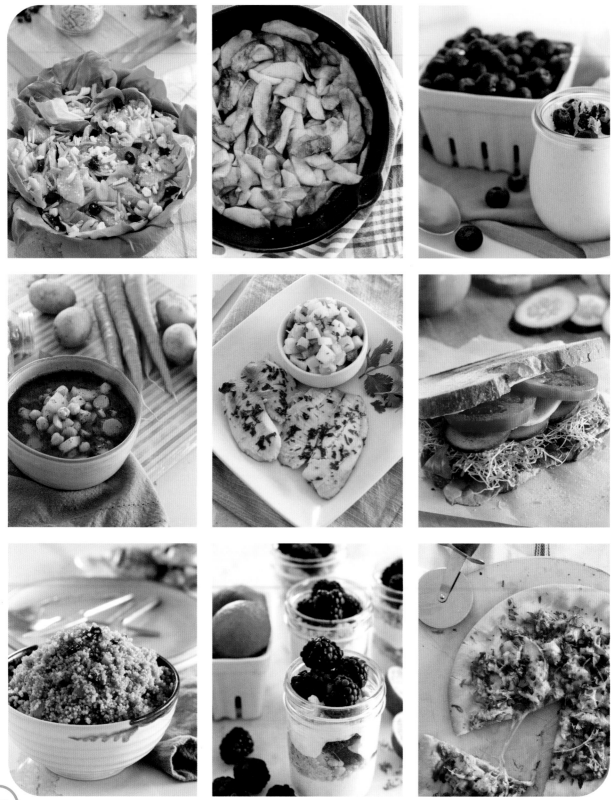

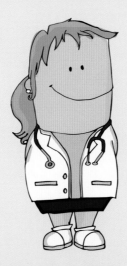

SECTION II

REINTRODUCTION, STEP BY STEP

In section II of this book, I will completely break down each stage of reintroduction one at a time. You will learn the suggested foods to eat for each challenge and their correct portion sizes to get accurate results without triggering a serious flare. I will share additional tips and customized recipes to help you enjoy the process. Lastly, I will discuss the final phase of the low-FODMAP diet: integration and personalization. By the end, you will have everything you need to successfully move forward with your personalized low-FODMAP lifestyle.

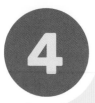

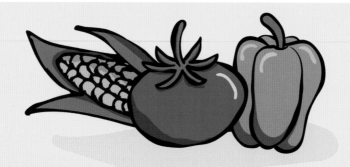

REINTRODUCTION, STAGE 1
FRUCTOSE, LACTOSE, SORBITOL, AND MANNITOL

FRUCTOSE

Fructose is a sugar classified as a *monosaccharide*. That means it is made up of one sugar group. Fructose can be also combined ("bound") with glucose to form a *disaccharide* known as sucrose, a.k.a. table sugar. Sucrose is more easily absorbed than fructose and is not high FODMAP, although it *can* irritate the gut in people with IBS.

"Excess fructose" is the high-FODMAP fructose that you will hear me referring to in this section. It is the fructose molecule that is NOT bound to glucose and is restricted during the elimination phase.

There are two types of intolerances to fructose. One is hereditary, meaning people are born with it. This is usually diagnosed soon after birth. The other intolerance is acquired later in life and is due to *malabsorption* of fructose, which is commonly seen with IBS.

For reasons we don't understand, certain individuals do not absorb fructose in their small intestine as quickly as others. Instead, the unabsorbed fructose is rapidly propelled into the colon, where it is fermented, leading to gas, bloating, and diarrhea.

The point of this challenge is to learn exactly how much fructose your body is capable of absorbing. This is going to be the running theme of all the challenges: Can I eat it, and if so, how much?

The challenges I outline below will have you consuming increasing amounts of excess fructose for three days in a row, followed by three break days, as outlined in chapter 2.

To test fructose, I recommended using honey, mango, or asparagus. The correct portion sizes to test for each of these foods are below.

HONEY

+ **Day 1: 10 g, about 1½ teaspoons**
+ **Day 2: 14 g, about 2 teaspoons**
+ **Day 3: 28 g, about 1 tablespoon**

MANGO

+ **Day 1: 52 g, about ¼ mango**
+ **Day 2: 104 g, about ½ mango**
+ **Day 3: 208 g, about 1 mango**

ASPARAGUS

+ **Day 1: 15 g, about 1 spear**
+ **Day 2: 30 g, about 2 spears**
+ **Day 3: 75 g, about 5 spears**

Remember to follow the low-FODMAP diet for three days after completing the challenges. Check out the sample weekly meal plan on page 111 for an example of how to incorporate this challenge into your weekly diet. You can use this as a template for the challenges going forward.

Once you've decided which food to test, you can choose to enjoy these foods on their own or try one of my suggested recipes. If you do enjoy the food alone, I suggest eating it during mealtime to best replicate your future behavior.

Remember, to get the best results, I recommend sticking to the same test food for all three days. Changing foods midway through the challenges could result in not escalating the amount appropriately, which could skew your findings.

Some great ways to enjoy honey include drizzling it on a piece of low-FODMAP toast with peanut butter, mixing it into your overnight oats or smoothie, adding it as a topping to your low-FODMAP yogurt and fruit, or stirring it into a cup of tea.

If you're planning to test asparagus, I highly recommend subbing it into my Crispy Cauliflower Tempura (page 125) or dressing it with my Balsamic and Rosemary Browned Butter (page 157).

To test mango, I've got a couple of great recipes for you to try: Simple Tropical Salad with Spinach (page 114) or Seared Tilapia with Mango Salsa (page 113).

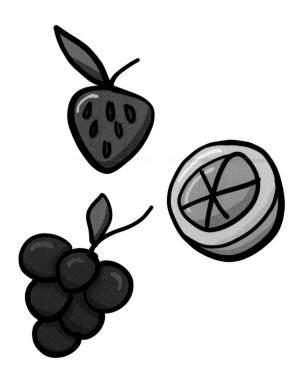

FIGURE 3. SAMPLE WEEKLY MEAL PLAN: FRUCTOSE

Fructose Challenge	Breakfast	Snack (optional)	Lunch	Snack or Dessert	Dinner
DAY 1 (break day: maintenance diet)	"Speculoos Cookie" Toasted Overnight Oats, page 47	Mandarin orange, sliced	Easy Caprese Panini, page 54	Irresistible Pumpkin-Spiced Granola, page 104	Turkey Taco Skillet, page 64
DAY 2 (break day: maintenance diet)	Carrot Cake Breakfast Cookies, page 40	1 cup (235 g) lactose-free yogurt and ⅓ medium banana	Leftover Turkey Taco Skillet, page 64	"Key Lime" Loaf, 1 slice, page 88	Brown Sugar–Glazed Meatloaf (page 66) with mashed potatoes
DAY 3 (break day: maintenance diet)	Homemade Cinnamon Crunch Bagel (page 45) and sliced orange	4 low-FODMAP crackers with 2 slices mozzarella cheese	Shrimp Sushi Bowl, page 57	"Oatstanding" Oatmeal, Chocolate, and Peanut Butter Cookie, page 95	Cheesy Chicken Pasta Bake, page 87
DAY 4 (Challenge Day 1)	Chocolate, Peanut Butter, and Banana Smoothie, page 44	1 medium carrot and ⅓ medium common cucumber, chopped	Denver Sandwich (page 50) with ¼ sliced mango (52 g)	4 low-FODMAP crackers with 1 tablespoon (15 g) almond butter	Orange Marmalade Salmon (page 83), baked potatoes, and green beans
DAY 5 (Challenge Day 2)	Low-FODMAP rice crisp cereal with lactose-free milk and ½ unripe banana	Irresistible Pumpkin-Spiced Granola, page 104	Simple Tropical Salad with Spinach, page 114	"Oatstanding" Oatmeal, Chocolate, and Peanut Butter Cookie, page 95	Lemon Parmesan Chicken Piccata (page 76) with low-FODMAP capellini
DAY 6 (Challenge Day 3)	Chai-Spiced French Toast (page 43) with maple syrup	1 ounce (28 g) roasted, salted peanuts	Seared Tilapia with Mango Salsa, page 113	"Key Lime" Loaf, 1 slice, page 88	Skillet Cottage Pie, page 75
DAY 7 (break day: maintenance diet)	"Hummingbird" Baked Oatmeal Bars, page 48	2 cups (16 g) popcorn	Leftover Skillet Cottage Pie, page 75	Decadent Chocolate Raspberry Mug Cake, page 102	Sheet Pan Orange Chicken with Broccoli, page 71
DAY 8 (break day: maintenance diet)	Zesty Greek Omelet, page 39	10 almonds	Leftover Sheet Pan Orange Chicken with Broccoli, page 71	"Oatstanding" Oatmeal, Chocolate, and Peanut Butter Cookie, page 95	Stir-Fry Ginger Shrimp and Vegetables (page 80) with steamed rice
DAY 9 (break day: maintenance diet)	Carrot Cake Breakfast Cookies, page 40	½ cup (120 g) lactose-free cottage cheese with 65 g chopped strawberries	Chicken Noodle Soup for One, page 51	Glazed Pineapple Walnut Muffin, page 101	Slow Cooker Vegan Sloppy Joes, page 79

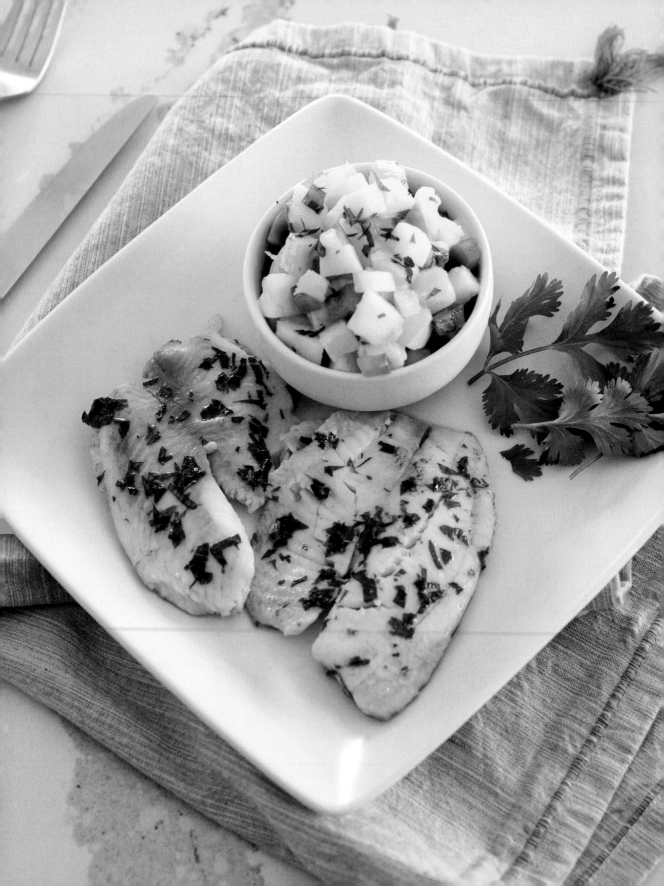

SEARED TILAPIA WITH MANGO SALSA

The flavor of mango is the perfect complement to a flaky and tender fish fillet. Tilapia is one of the most affordable fish choices, and a healthy one as well. It is low in calories, high in protein, and filled with omega-3 fats and important nutrients. FODMAP fact: Green and red bell peppers vary in their FODMAP content. Red bell peppers are higher in FODMAPs (per gram) due to fructose, while green bell peppers in excess contain fructans. Don't take anything for granted with FODMAPs!

To make the tilapia: In a shallow bowl or resealable bag, whisk together the infused oil, lemon juice, parsley, basil, pepper, and salt. Place the tilapia in the bowl or bag and seal well. Refrigerate for 1 hour to marinate.

To make the mango salsa: While the fish is marinating, prepare your mango salsa by combining the pineapple (if using), bell pepper, and cilantro. Add the lime and lemon juices and toss well to combine. Separate the salsa into two portions, and allocate the mango to each one per the noted portion sizes. Store the salsa in the refrigerator until the fish is ready to serve.

Once the fish is fully marinated, heat the canola oil in a large cast-iron skillet over medium heat. Remove the tilapia from the marinade and discard the liquid. Place the fillets in your skillet and sear on both sides until the fish is fully cooked through, 3 to 4 minutes per side. Serve the tilapia with the mango salsa and additional cilantro leaves.

VARIATION: To make this recipe suitable for the FODMAP elimination phase, use 360 g of fresh fruit: 280 g pineapple and 80 g of mango for 2 servings.

FOR THE SEARED TILAPIA:

¼ cup (60 ml) garlic-infused oil

1 tablespoon (15 ml) lemon juice

1 tablespoon (4 g) minced fresh parsley

1 teaspoon dried basil

1 teaspoon ground black pepper

½ teaspoon salt

2 (6-ounce [168 g]) tilapia fillets

1 tablespoon (15 ml) canola or avocado oil, for cooking

Salt and pepper to taste

FOR THE MANGO SALSA:

About 400 g mix of fresh ripe mango and fresh pineapple, peeled and chopped into small chunks; adjust portion based on day of challenge:

+ **Day 1: 52 g mango per serving (104 g total) and 140 g pineapple per serving (280 g total)**

+ **Day 2: 104 g mango per serving (208 g total) and 100 g pineapple per serving (200 g total)**

+ **Day 3: 208 g mango per serving (416 g total, about 2 mangoes); omit pineapple**

½ green bell pepper (50 g), diced

1 tablespoon (1 g) chopped fresh cilantro, plus more for garnish

2 tablespoons (30 ml) fresh lime juice (½ lime)

1 tablespoon (15 ml) fresh lemon juice

NUTRITION PER SERVING (DAY 1): Serving Size: 428 g, Calories: 410, Total Fat: 19 g, Saturated Fat: 2.5 g, Carbohydrates: 30 g, Sugar: 22 g, Sodium: 270 mg, Fiber: 3 g, Protein: 35 g

SIMPLE TROPICAL SALAD WITH SPINACH

A light and flavorful salad that incorporates fresh tropical fruits, spinach, and roasted peanuts. In this recipe, you are using mango as your fructose test food. You will increase the portion of mango in the recipe depending on the day of the challenge. The mango is deliciously paired with pineapple, which is a low-FODMAP fruit that you can enjoy in servings up to 140 g.

FOR THE DRESSING:

Juice of 1 medium lime (about 3 tablespoons [45 ml])

1 tablespoon (15 ml) olive oil

1 tablespoon (12 g) sugar

¼ teaspoon mustard powder

¼ teaspoon poppy seeds

FOR THE SALAD:

1 cup (50 g) torn baby spinach leaves

¼ (100 g) common cucumber, sliced into crescents

About 200 g mix of fresh ripe mango and fresh pineapple, peeled and chopped into small chunks; adjust portion based on day of challenge:

+ **Day 1: 52 g mango and 140 g pineapple**

+ **Day 2: 104 g mango and 100 g pineapple**

+ **Day 3: 208 g mango (no pineapple)**

1 tablespoon (6 g) chopped scallions, green tips only, or chives

Salt and pepper to taste

FOR THE GARNISH:

2 tablespoons (15 g) roasted salted peanuts

To make the dressing: Whisk all the dressing ingredients in a small cup or bowl.

To make the salad: In a medium bowl, combine the spinach, cucumber, mango, pineapple, and scallions. Season with salt and pepper, then drizzle with the desired amount of dressing. Toss everything together, then garnish with the peanuts before serving.

VARIATION: To make this recipe suitable for the FODMAP elimination phase, use 180 g of fresh fruit: 140 g pineapple and 40 g of mango.

TIP: To chop a mango, slice it in half and remove the stone. Then, using your knife, cut horizontal and vertical lines in each half, transecting each other to form a grid. Then, simply fold the peel backward and spoon out each individual piece. It works like a charm.

NUTRITION PER SERVING (DAY 1): Serving Size: 436 g, Calories: 400, Total Fat: 23 g, Saturated Fat: 3.5 g, Carbohydrates: 49 g, Sugar: 35 g, Sodium: 90 mg, Fiber: 7 g, Protein: 8 g

LACTOSE

Lactose is a disaccharide, a sugar formed by binding two sugars together. In the case of lactose, those two sugars are galactose and glucose.

Lactose is absorbed in our small intestines by a specific enzyme known as *lactase*. The production of this enzyme can decline with age and other factors, leading to malabsorption.

Lactose intolerance typically causes a more severe digestive response to lactose than the sensitivity seen with IBS. Milk protein allergy is another phenomenon, related to the proteins in milk, rather than lactose. If you are lactose intolerant, or have a milk allergy, you should omit this challenge. I recommend you skip to the next section to continue.

Lactose is commonly found in milk and milk products, and those are the products you will be testing in this FODMAP category. To test lactose, I recommend using cow's milk, cow's milk yogurt, or ricotta cheese. You can substitute some cow's milk or yogurt for your usual low-FODMAP brand in your favorite smoothie, oats, or other recipe. My Chocolate, Peanut Butter, and Banana Smoothie (page 44) or my Grapefruit-Orange Julius (page 131) are great options for this. If you want to use ricotta, options include enjoying a small amount on a cracker with some fruit or stirring some into your morning scrambled eggs for extra creaminess.

Whichever you choose, make sure you're consuming the correct amount of lactose each challenge day. The correct portion sizes to test lactose using cow's milk, cow's milk yogurt, or ricotta cheese are:

COW'S MILK (NONFAT, 1%, 2%):

+ **Day 1: ¼ cup (62 ml)**

+ **Day 2: ½ cup (125 ml)**

+ **Day 3: 1 cup (250 ml)**

PLAIN COW'S MILK YOGURT:

+ **Day 1: 85 g, about 3 ounces**

+ **Day 2: 170 g, about 6 ounces**

+ **Day 3: 200 g, about 7 ounces**

RICOTTA CHEESE:

+ **Day 1: 50 g, about 1.7 ounces**

+ **Day 2: 80 g, about 2.8 ounces**

+ **Day 3: 120 g, about 4.25 ounces**

Remember to follow the low-FODMAP diet for three days after completing the challenges.

Following are some recipes for you to try.

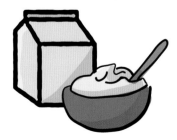

SUNNY LEMON YOGURT WITH BLUEBERRIES

Adding citrus to plain yogurt makes for a tart, tasty treat. This recipe uses fresh lemon juice and zest, plus fresh berries to add a sweet note to the creamy snack. Not a fan of blueberries? Sub fresh strawberries or raspberries instead. A low-FODMAP serving of raspberries is 60 g, and strawberries is 65 g.

2 tablespoons (30 ml) lemon juice (½ lemon)

1 teaspoon lemon zest, plus more for garnish

227 g (about 1 cup) yogurt, mixture of cow's milk and lactose-free; adjust portion based on day of challenge:

+ **Day 1: 85 g (about 3 ounces) cow's milk yogurt and 142 g (about 5 ounces) lactose-free**

+ **Day 2: 170 g (about 6 ounces) cow's milk yogurt and 57 g (about 2 ounces) lactose-free**

+ **Day 3: 200 g (about 7 ounces) cow's milk yogurt and 27 g (about 1 ounce) lactose-free**

¼ teaspoon vanilla extract

2 tablespoons (25 g) sugar

1½ ounces (40 g) fresh blueberries

In a medium bowl, whisk together the lemon juice, zest, and yogurt. Add the vanilla and sugar. Top with fresh blueberries and additional lemon zest.

VARIATION: To make this suitable for the FODMAP elimination phase, use all lactose-free yogurt.

NOTES:
+ This yogurt does have a sweet flavor. If you prefer a less sweet variety, then adjust the sugar to your preference.

+ To make a sugar-free version of this recipe, substitute stevia or sucralose for the sugar.

NUTRITION PER SERVING (DAY 1): Serving Size: 326 g, Calories: 290, Total Fat: 8 g, Saturated Fat: 6 g, Carbohydrates: 47 g, Sugar: 39 g, Sodium: 105 mg, Fiber: 1 g, Protein: 8 g

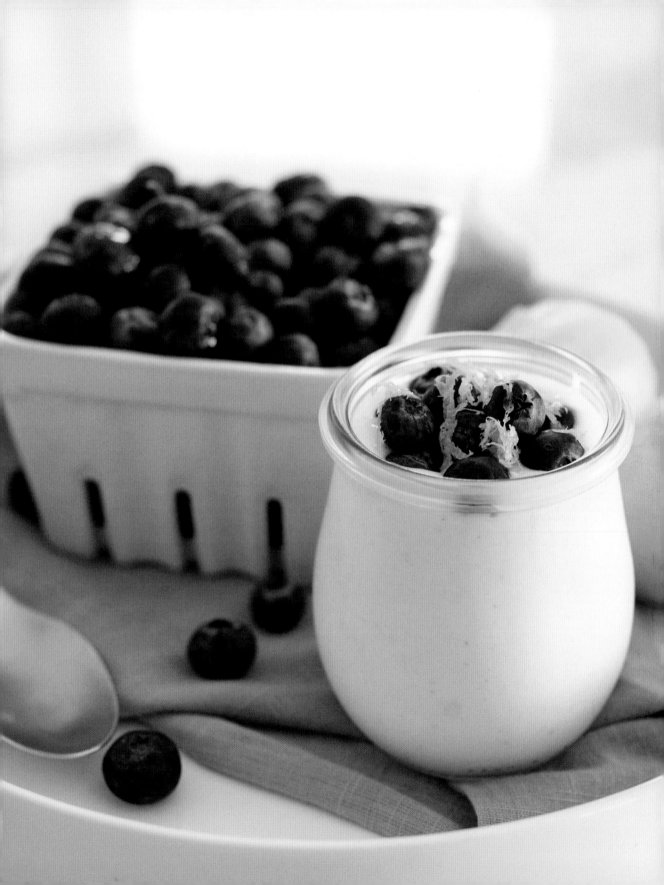

Yield: 1 serving   Prep time: 5 minutes

ENERGIZING COFFEE YOGURT

I used to love coffee yogurt, so I couldn't resist creating my own low-FODMAP version to enjoy now. The result is a snack that goes great with berries, toasted oats or nuts, low-FODMAP granola (see page 104), chocolate chips, or rice crisp cereal.

1 teaspoon instant espresso granules

½ teaspoon warm water

½ teaspoon vanilla extract

227 g (about 1 cup) yogurt, mixture of cow's milk and lactose-free; adjust portion based on day of challenge:

+ **Day 1: 85 g (about 3 ounces) cow's milk yogurt and 142 g (about 5 ounces) lactose-free**

+ **Day 2: 170 g (about 6 ounces) cow's milk yogurt and 57 g (about 2 ounces) lactose-free**

+ **Day 3: 200 g (about 7 ounces) cow's milk yogurt and 27 g (about 1 ounce) lactose-free**

2 tablespoons (25 g) sugar

In a medium bowl, dissolve the espresso granules in the warm water and vanilla. Add the yogurt and stir thoroughly until the mixture is smooth. Mix in the sugar and enjoy!

VARIATION: To make this suitable for the FODMAP elimination phase, use all lactose-free yogurt.

NOTES:

+ This yogurt does have a sweet flavor. If you prefer a less sweet variety, then adjust the sugar to your preference.

+ To make a sugar-free version of this recipe, substitute stevia or sucralose for the sugar.

NUTRITION PER SERVING (DAY 1): Serving Size: 259 g, Calories: 270, Total Fat: 8 g, Saturated Fat: 6 g, Carbohydrates: 40 g, Sugar: 34 g, Sodium: 105 mg, Fiber: 0 g, Protein: 8 g

TUMMY-TAMING TECHNIQUES

These are my favorite techniques to manage IBS flares and reduce stress. You may find them useful as you move through the reintroduction phase of the FODMAP journey.

Belly Breathing

Stress is a common trigger for IBS. Here is a simple breathing exercise that helps release stress. This exercise uses a technique called *belly breathing*. Belly breathing expands your abdomen and soothes your gut.

Start by finding a comfortable seat or lying flat in a comfortable position. Place one hand on your belly just below your ribs and one hand on your chest. Take a deep breath in through your nose, and let your belly push your hand out. If you are doing it correctly, your chest should stay still. Breathe out through pursed lips as if you are whistling.

Gently breathe in and out in this manner three to ten times. Take your time with each breath.

After you have mastered belly breathing, try 4-7-8 breathing.

4-7-8 Breathing

This technique, called *4-7-8 breathing*, involves three timed intervals using belly breathing. This is how it works:

- Inhale from your belly, counting to 4 as you breathe in.

- At the top of the inhale, hold your breath while you count from 1 to 7.

- Slowly exhale while counting to 8, releasing all the air from your lungs.

Repeat this exercise at least three times or until you start to feel more relaxed. You can do it any time of day, whenever you need to balance your mental well-being.

Yoga

Yoga is a great way to improve IBS symptoms. The physical practice makes your body feel good, while the mindful practice eases stress and calms the nervous system.

There are five poses that are of the greatest help in reducing abdominal discomfort. For full details, see my blog post "Five Amazing Yoga Poses to Help Reduce IBS Symptoms" on my website at www.rachelpaulsfood.com. However, my favorite is Wind-Relieving Pose (Pavana Muktasana). This pose improves digestion and lengthens the spine. It also incorporates belly breathing. Here's how to do it:

Lying on your back, bring your right knee toward your chest, interlacing your fingers over your shin. Keep the other leg extended, but engaged, and your spine flat on a floor mat.

When you inhale, feel your belly expand into your right thigh, and with your exhale, pull your knee closer to your heart. This gives your digestive tract a gentle massage.

Take as many breaths as you like, then transition to the opposite side and repeat.

Abdominal Massage

Abdominal massage stimulates digestion and encourages gas passage or bowel movements.

Lie on your back with your knees gently bent over a rolled towel or pillow. This posture relaxes your abdominal wall muscles and allows the massage to penetrate deeper.

Place the palm of your hand on the lower right side of your belly. In a clockwise fashion, press up and around to the lower left side.

Repeat this motion slowly as many times as you desire.

POLYOLS: SORBITOL AND MANNITOL

Polyols (polyalcohols), also known as sugar alcohols, occur naturally in fruits and vegetables. They are also commonly added to commercial food products to create a sweet flavor with fewer calories. Sugar alcohols are slowly and incompletely absorbed in the small intestine, thus packing in an excessive amount leads to bloating and diarrhea.

The two polyalcohols that we will be challenging are sorbitol and mannitol. While they are both polyols, these two compounds vary in their chemical structure and sources in nature. Therefore, they are typically challenged separately, and reported individually in the Monash and FODMAP Friendly apps.

You may be aware of other polyols. One example, erythritol, is better absorbed in the small intestine and less associated with diarrhea and bloating. By contrast, xylitol (found in sugar-free gum and mints) can cause digestive upset in many individuals, not just people with IBS. I do not recommend challenging xylitol in this phase of reintroduction. If this was an important or beloved part of your pre-FODMAP diet, you can consider testing upon completion of all the challenges.

POLYOLS: SORBITOL

The first polyol challenge will be sorbitol. As with the other stage 1 challenges, begin testing after three break days.

The recommended test foods for sorbitol are avocado, blackberries, and yellow peaches (ONLY yellow peaches; other varieties may contain higher levels or different subgroups of FODMAPs). These test foods are easy to enjoy on their own: Try slicing some avocado on your usual lunchtime salad or sandwich or add a few blackberries to your morning yogurt. If you want something a little more put together, I have some great recipes for you.

See the list on the right for the recommended portion sizes for testing sorbitol using avocado, blackberries, or yellow peaches.

AVOCADO:
+ **Day 1: 40 g, about ¼ small**
+ **Day 2: 80 g, about ½ small**
+ **Day 3: 120 g, about ¾ medium**

BLACKBERRIES:
+ **Day 1: 13 g, about 2 or 3 berries**
+ **Day 2: 25 g, about 5 berries**
+ **Day 3: 50 g, about 10 berries**

YELLOW PEACHES:
+ **Day 1: 37 g, about ¼ peach**
+ **Day 2: 73 g, about ½ peach**
+ **Day 3: 146 g, about 1 peach**

Remember to follow the low-FODMAP diet for three days after completing the challenges and record your symptoms in your journal.

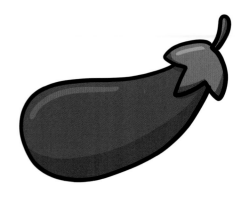

PERFECT AVOCADO TOAST

Avocado toast is a food trend I'm thrilled to participate in. I've always been a fan of mashing avocado with a little lemon, salt, and oil and spreading it on crusty bread. Since you have complete control over the amount of avocado you use, it's the perfect recipe for testing sorbitol, or just enjoying avocado for its own sake.

In a small bowl, mash the avocado. Add the lemon juice, salt, and pepper and mix well. Toast your slice(s) of bread and top with the avocado mixture. Drizzle with oil and sprinkle with additional salt, pumpkin seeds, and feta, if desired.

NOTE: For the best avocado toast, ingredient quality is key. Use a hearty low-FODMAP bread, good-quality olive oil, and toast your pumpkin seeds to bring out their flavor (see Note, page 48).

Avocado, ripe; adjust portion based on day of challenge:

+ **Day 1: 40 g, about ¼ small avocado**

+ **Day 2: 80 g, about ½ small avocado**

+ **Day 3: 120 g, about ¾ medium avocado**

½ teaspoon fresh lemon juice

⅛ teaspoon kosher salt

⅛ teaspoon freshly ground black pepper

1 or 2 slices low-FODMAP, gluten-free bread of your choice or sourdough (see "FODMAP FAQs," page 20)

½ to 1 teaspoon extra-virgin olive oil

Optional toppings: sea salt flakes, toasted pumpkin seeds (pepitas), crumbled feta cheese (omit for vegan version)

NUTRITION PER SERVING (DAY 1): Serving Size: 74 g, Calories: 150, Total Fat: 10 g, Saturated Fat: 1.5 g, Carbohydrates: 17 g, Sugar: 1 g, Sodium: 370 mg, Fiber: 3 g, Protein: 2 g

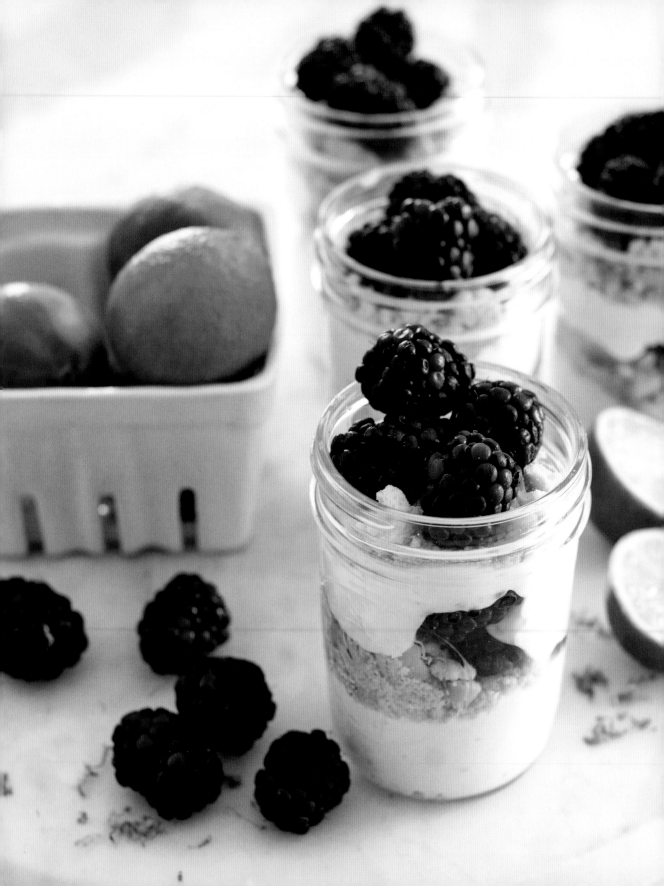

LIME CUSTARD TRIFLES WITH BLACKBERRIES

This is a dessert you will enjoy serving to your fanciest guests. It's a no-bake recipe that results in a rich and creamy lime custard, layered with cookie crumbles and fresh berries. Served individually in mason jars or parfait glasses, these trifles look so elegant, no one will guess how easy they are.

In a small heavy saucepan over medium-low heat, whisk the egg yolks, 6 tablespoons (75 g) of the sugar, and lime juice until blended, about 1 minute. Keep a close eye on this, adjusting the heat as necessary; do not let it burn. Add the butter, whisking constantly until the mixture has thickened and coats the back of a spoon, about 4 minutes. Remove the pan from the heat and stir in the lime zest and extract. Transfer the curd to a small bowl to cool slightly. Cover the bowl with plastic wrap, tucking the wrap inside the bowl so it lays completely flat on the surface of the curd. Refrigerate until chilled, at least 1 hour.

When your curd is chilled, toss your berries with the remaining 1 teaspoon of sugar in a separate small bowl, and set aside in the refrigerator. In a large bowl with an electric mixer, beat the heavy cream until thickened, 1 to 2 minutes. Turn your mixer down to low and add the chilled lime curd, beating to incorporate, then increase the mixer to high and beat until medium peaks form.

Spoon half of the whipped lime custard into four mason jars or parfait glasses. Top with half of the cookie crumbs and half the blackberries. Repeat these layers with the remaining curd and crumbs, topping the entire trifle with the remaining blackberries. Serve immediately or keep in the fridge for 2 to 3 days.

VARIATIONS:

+ Substitute lemon for the lime and enjoy lemon custard trifles instead.

+ To enjoy this recipe on the FODMAP elimination phase, use strawberries in place of blackberries.

NOTE: This trifle is wonderful with both chocolate and vanilla cookie crumbles.

3 egg yolks

6 tablespoons (75 g) plus 1 teaspoon sugar, divided

¼ cup (60 ml) fresh lime juice (about 2 limes)

¼ cup (56 g) unsalted butter

2 teaspoons finely grated lime zest

¼ teaspoon lime extract

6 ounces (170 g) fresh blackberries; adjust personal portion based on day of challenge:

+ **Day 1: 13 g, 2 or 3 berries**

+ **Day 2: 25 g, 5 berries**

+ **Day 3: 50 g, 10 berries**

¾ cup (180 ml) heavy whipping cream

4 ounces (120 g, or about 8) low-FODMAP, gluten-free cookies of your choice, crushed

NUTRITION PER SERVING*: Serving Size: 152 g, Calories: 530, Total Fat: 36 g, Saturated Fat: 21 g, Carbohydrates: 47 g, Sugar: 36 g, Sodium: 85 mg, Fiber: 1 g, Protein: 5 g

* Nutritional analysis for this recipe is calculated based on the standard serving size, *not* the recommended portion for FODMAP reintroduction testing.

POLYOLS: MANNITOL

Unlike sorbitol, mannitol is commonly found in vegetables. The recommended test foods for mannitol are cauliflower, celery, and sweet potato.

This is another challenge where the test foods can be easily enjoyed on their own. I love celery stalks spread with peanut butter, or raw cauliflower with a bit of ranch dressing. Cauliflower is also delicious steamed with some grated Cheddar cheese. If testing sweet potato, you can't go wrong with a baked sweet potato topped with butter and cinnamon. Alternatively, try one of my following recipes.

The recommended portion sizes for testing mannitol using cauliflower, celery, or sweet potato are listed on the right.

CAULIFLOWER:

+ **Day 1: 17 g, about 2 florets**

+ **Day 2: 33 g, about 4 florets**

+ **Day 3: 66 g, about 8 florets**

CELERY:

+ **Day 1: 19 g, about ½ medium stalk**

+ **Day 2: 38 g, about 1 medium stalk**

+ **Day 3: 60 g, about 1 large stalk**

SWEET POTATO (RAW WEIGHT):

+ **Day 1: 105 g, about ¾ cup**

+ **Day 2: 140 g, about 1 cup**

+ **Day 3: 210 g, about 1½ cups**

Don't forget to follow the low-FODMAP diet for three days after completing the challenges.

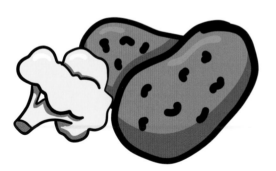

Planning on using raw veggies for this challenge? Try dipping them in my homemade ranch dressing, recipe on page 58!

CRISPY CAULIFLOWER TEMPURA WITH SESAME MUSTARD DIPPING SAUCE

This gluten-free tempura recipe is guaranteed to be your new favorite for all your veggies. A light and crispy batter makes everything taste better. Don't forget the dipping sauce, the ideal accompaniment for this healthy Asian dish.

To make the dipping sauce: Combine all the sauce ingredients in a small bowl and set aside.

To make the tempura: Line a plate with paper towels. In a large bowl, whisk the club soda, rice flour, and salt until well combined. Dip the cauliflower in the batter, tapping off any excess, and transfer to a plate.

Set a large pan over high heat and fill with about 3 inches (7.5 cm) of oil. Use a cooking thermometer to heat the oil to 350°F (180°C), or gas mark 4. Working with a few pieces at a time to maintain the oil temperature, fry the tempura in the oil for 1 to 2 minutes on each side until lightly browned. Use metal tongs to transfer the tempura to the pan and slightly stir each piece in the oil. Watch them carefully so they don't burn. Remove the cauliflower pieces with a slotted spoon to the prepared plate. Season with salt to taste and serve with the dipping sauce on the side.

*Make sure your brand does not contain high-fructose corn syrup.

VARIATION: Try this with sliced carrots, parsnips, potatoes, zucchini, and yellow squash to make it suitable for the FODMAP elimination phase.

FOR THE SESAME MUSTARD DIPPING SAUCE:

1 teaspoon mustard powder

2 tablespoons (30 ml) mirin*

2 teaspoons soy sauce, gluten-free if necessary

1 teaspoon toasted sesame oil

½ teaspoon rice vinegar

1 tablespoon (15 ml) maple syrup

FOR THE TEMPURA:

⅓ cup (80 ml) cold club soda

⅓ cup (40 g) finely ground white rice flour

¼ teaspoon salt, plus to taste

1 cup (about 100 g) chopped cauliflower; adjust personal portion based on day of challenge:

+ **Day 1: 17 g, about 2 florets**

+ **Day 2: 33 g, about 4 florets**

+ **Day 3: 66 g, about 8 florets**

Canola or other high smoke point oil, for frying

NUTRITION PER SERVING**: Serving Size: 67 g, Calories: 80, Total Fat: 2 g, Saturated Fat: 0 g, Carbohydrates: 16 g, Sugar: 6 g, Sodium: 370 mg, Fiber: 1 g, Protein: 2 g

** Nutritional analysis for this recipe is calculated based on the standard serving size, *not* the recommended portion for FODMAP reintroduction testing.

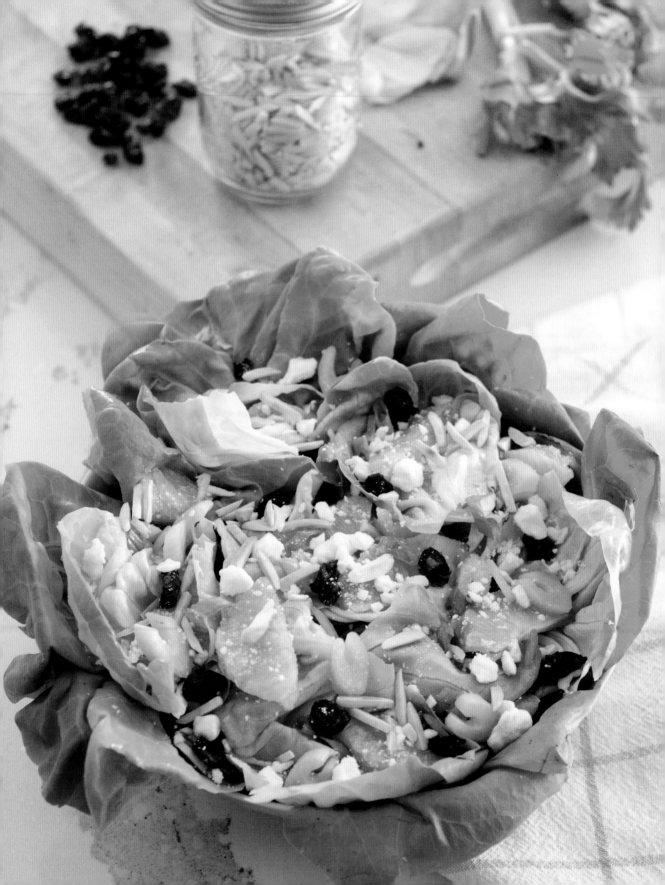

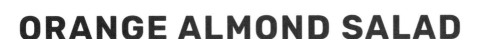

ORANGE ALMOND SALAD

The flavors of orange and almond are a lovely combination in this sweet salad recipe. My mother used to serve an orange almond salad at every fancy occasion. Adding dried cranberries and feta makes it even more special.

To make the dressing: In a small bowl, whisk the dressing ingredients.

To make the salad: In a large bowl, combine the lettuce, scallion tips, and orange pieces. Drizzle the dressing over the salad and toss to coat. Plate the salads, then add in the designated amount of celery to each portion. Sprinkle everything with the toasted almonds, cranberries, and feta, if using.

VARIATION: To make this recipe suitable for the FODMAP elimination phase, consume 10 g of celery per serving.

NOTE: Canned oranges have not been tested for FODMAP content. Do not substitute canned mandarins in this recipe.

FOR THE DRESSING:

2 tablespoons (30 ml) olive or canola oil

1 tablespoon (12 g) sugar

1 teaspoon Dijon mustard

2 tablespoons (30 ml) freshly squeezed orange juice

1 tablespoon (15 ml) red wine vinegar

Salt and pepper to taste

FOR THE SALAD:

1½ cups (120 g) torn Bibb or butter lettuce

2 scallions, green tips only, chopped

1 large navel orange or 3 clementines/mandarins (200 g), peeled and separated into wedges, pith removed

2 medium stalks celery (80 g), chopped; adjust personal portion based on day of challenge:

+ **Day 1: 19 g, about ½ medium stalk**

+ **Day 2: 38 g, about 1 medium stalk**

+ **Day 3: 60 g, about 1 large stalk**

2 teaspoons (15 g) toasted sliced or slivered almonds

2 tablespoons (20 g) dried cranberries

¼ cup (25 g) crumbled feta cheese (omit for vegan version)

* Nutritional analysis for this recipe is calculated based on the standard serving size, *not* the recommended portion for FODMAP reintroduction testing.

NUTRITION PER SERVING*: Serving Size: 234 g, Calories: 280, Total Fat: 18 g, Saturated Fat: 4 g, Carbohydrates: 29 g, Sugar: 22 g, Sodium: 210 mg, Fiber: 4 g, Protein: 4 g

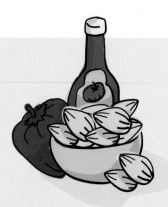

REINTRODUCTION, STAGE 2
FRUCTANS AND GALACTANS (GOS)

FRUCTANS

You have probably noticed that testing fructans will require a few weeks. This is because fructans are a very complex type of FODMAP.

Fructans include the subtypes fructo-oligosaccharides (FOS), oligofructose, and inulins. Their classification is based on their chemical composition—specifically, the number of sugars in the fructan molecule. Fructans with shorter chains are fermented more quickly; these include onions and garlic. Inulins are fructans that have longer chain lengths; these include chicory root and Jerusalem artichokes.

Generally speaking, humans don't have enough of the essential enzymes necessary to break apart the linkages connecting the chains. As a result, only about 5 to 15 percent of the chains are absorbed in the small intestine. The remaining fructans continue on to the large bowel, where they are fermented. This creates water movement into the gut, and consequently diarrhea, discomfort, and bloating. As you have learned, these symptoms are more uncomfortable if you have IBS.

To simplify their data, the Monash and FODMAP Friendly apps do not separate out the fructan subtypes in their reports. However, foods often contain multiple different fructans. They are found in variable food groups, including fruits, vegetables, and grains.

Because of their complexity, fructans require more extensive testing than other FODMAPs. Therefore, we will test the fructan group using four categories. You are going to do the fruit and vegetable category first, followed by wheat, then onion, and finally, garlic. Some individuals with IBS react uniquely to garlic, compared with other fructans, so it gets a special category all on its own.

If this sounds like a lot of work, don't worry. Remember, it's not a race. The important thing is to do things right. This schedule, while a little time-consuming, will provide you with more accurate results and will minimize discomfort.

You have now finished all four stage 1 challenges. That's halfway through all the standard FODMAP categories. Amazing work so far! The next several challenges are for fructans and galactans (GOS). For these categories, I recommend having a test day separated by a "break" or "washout" day. This provides extra time for the foods you're testing to make it through your system, because these options tend to digest more slowly than the previous FODMAP foods.

FRUCTANS: FRUITS AND VEGETABLES

The recommended test foods for the first category of fructans, fruits and vegetables, are grapefruit, raisins, and Brussels sprouts. You can enjoy a grapefruit cut in half as a side to your breakfast, sprinkle raisins over your salad, or steam Brussels sprouts for your supper. I also have some great recipes for you to try.

If you have issues tolerating high-acid foods due to gut sensitivity or acid reflux (GERD), I suggest avoiding grapefruit as your challenge food. It could aggravate your symptoms.

The correct portion sizes for testing grapefruit, raisins, or Brussels sprouts for the first fructan challenge are as follows:

GRAPEFRUIT:

+ **Day 1: 104 g, about ½ medium**

+ **Day 2: break day**

+ **Day 3: 207 g, about 1 medium**

+ **Day 4: break day**

+ **Day 5: 280 g, about 1 large**

+ **Day 6: break day**

RAISINS:

+ **Day 1: 19 g, about 1½ tablespoons**

+ **Day 2: break day**

+ **Day 3: 26 g, about 2 tablespoons**

+ **Day 4: break day**

+ **Day 5: 39 g, about 3 tablespoons**

+ **Day 6: break day**

BRUSSELS SPROUTS (RAW WEIGHT):

+ **Day 1: 57 g, about 3 sprouts**

+ **Day 2: break day**

+ **Day 3: 76 g, about 4 sprouts**

+ **Day 4: break day**

+ **Day 5: 95 g, about 5 sprouts**

+ **Day 6: break day**

You are doing so well! I know this seems like a long process, but you have come so far. Stick to it. You only have a few more categories to go!

GRAPEFRUIT-ORANGE JULIUS

This refreshing smoothie is packed with flavor and health benefits. While similar to the "Orange Julius" from my childhood shopping-mall kiosk, this beverage is made using fresh, natural ingredients. Be sure to get all the pith off the grapefruit to eliminate any bitterness (see Tip, below). FODMAP fact: Although both are citrus fruits, grapefruit contains fructans while navel oranges in excess contain fructose. Don't take anything for granted with FODMAPs!

Place all the ingredients, except the sugar and milk, in a blender and blend well on high. Taste and add sugar and milk as desired. Serve immediately.

VARIATION: Use 80 g grapefruit and 150 g navel orange to enjoy this during the FODMAP elimination phase.

TIP: Sectioning a grapefruit is a bit tricky, but the pith will make it taste bitter if you don't remove it all. I found it easiest to slice the fruit in half over a bowl, then cut around each triangle of flesh and remove them, then squeeze all the juice and flesh off the rind.

About 280 g mix of ripe grapefruit and navel orange, peeled and sectioned, pith removed (include all the juice); adjust portion based on day of challenge:

+ **Day 1: 104 g grapefruit and 150 g navel orange**

+ **Day 3: 207 g grapefruit and 83 g navel orange**

+ **Day 5: 280 g grapefruit only**

⅓ cup (80 g) ice

¼ cup (60 g) low-FODMAP plain yogurt, such as lactose-free or coconut for vegan version

1 teaspoon vanilla extract

1 to 2 tablespoons (12 to 24 g) sugar

1 to 2 tablespoons low-FODMAP milk, such as lactose-free or almond milk, optional, for consistency

NUTRITION PER SERVING (DAY 1): Serving Size: 425 g, Calories: 230, Total Fat: 2.5 g, Saturated Fat: 1.5 g, Carbohydrates: 47 g, Sugar: 35 g, Sodium: 40 mg, Fiber: 5 g, Protein: 5 g

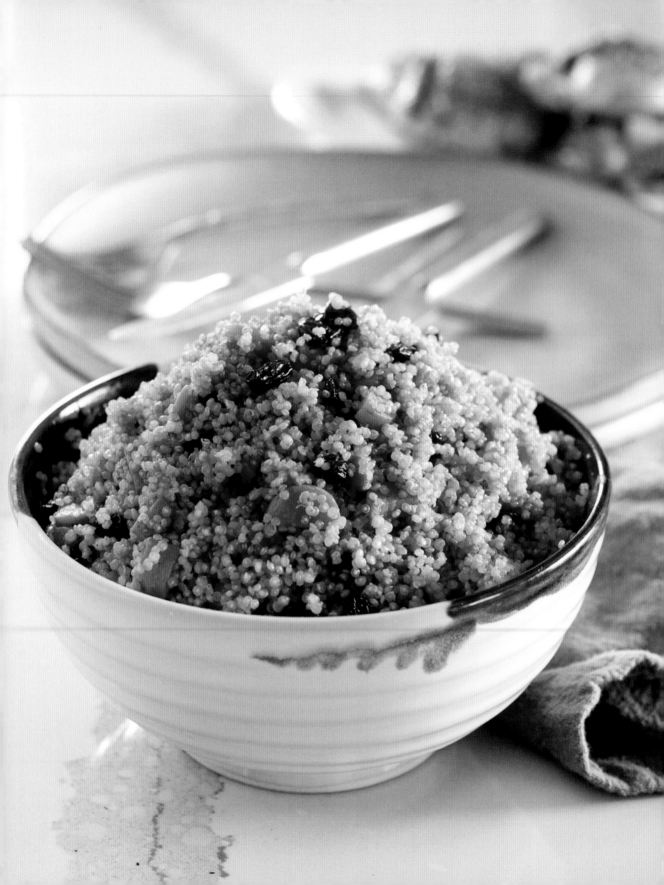

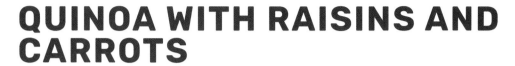
QUINOA WITH RAISINS AND CARROTS

This quinoa is a hit with my whole family. The flavors of curry and cinnamon, combined with carrots and sweet raisins, reminds me of Moroccan and Indian cuisines. It's a side dish that goes beautifully with any roasted chicken, beef, or fish entrée.

1 cup (173 g) uncooked quinoa, rinsed

1½ cups (355 ml) low-FODMAP vegan stock or broth, gluten-free if necessary (see Note, page 61)

¼ cup (30 g) chopped carrots

¼ teaspoon salt

1 tablespoon (15 ml) olive or avocado oil

½ teaspoon curry powder*

⅛ teaspoon ground cinnamon

½ cup (80 g) raisins; adjust personal portion based on day of challenge:

+ **Day 1: 19 g, about 1½ tablespoons**

+ **Day 3: 26 g, about 2 tablespoons**

+ **Day 5: 39 g, about 3 tablespoons**

Combine the quinoa, stock, carrots, salt, oil, and spices in a medium saucepan. Cover and cook over medium heat for about 15 minutes or until all the water is absorbed and the quinoa is tender. Stir the quinoa to fluff it, and taste to adjust the seasoning as needed. Divide among four bowls and stir raisins into each portion before serving.

*Some curry powders contain added onion and garlic. Check your brand to make sure it is low FODMAP.

VARIATION: To make this suitable for the FODMAP elimination phase, limit the raisin portion to 13 g per serving.

NUTRITION PER SERVING****:** Serving Size: 164 g, Calories: 250, Total Fat: 6 g, Saturated Fat: 1 g, Carbohydrates: 44 g, Sugar: 14 g, Sodium: 310 mg, Fiber: 4 g, Protein: 7 g

** Nutritional analysis for this recipe is calculated based on the standard serving size, *not* the recommended portion for FODMAP reintroduction testing.

FRUCTANS: WHEAT

The second fructan challenge is the wheat/grain challenge. This is a challenge that you should omit if you are gluten intolerant or have celiac disease. It is also one to pass over if you have non-celiac gluten sensitivity.

Many people incorrectly assume that the low-FODMAP diet is a gluten-free diet. You already know that it is not! FODMAPs are carbohydrates, while gluten is a protein. The symptoms people experience after consuming grain-containing foods are caused by the fructans in wheat and barley. Gluten is often just an innocent bystander.

If you tolerate these challenges, that's awesome! You may be able to add wheat-containing foods back into your diet. Just be aware that some breads and other grain products may contain high-fructose corn syrup, inulin, and high-FODMAP additives. Always check your ingredient list to ensure you are not accidentally consuming FODMAPs (see "How to Read Labels," page 26).

The suggested challenge foods for testing the wheat category of fructans are wheat pasta or white bread. Do not substitute wheat or multigrain breads here; those will be challenged later. You can enjoy the bread in your favorite sandwich or use my recipes for Easy Caprese Panini (page 54), Denver Sandwich (page 50), or Chai-Spiced French Toast (page 43). If you prefer pasta for this challenge, try my Chicken Noodle Soup for One (page 51). Or see more recipes on the following pages.

WHEAT PASTA, ANY TYPE (COOKED WEIGHT):

+ **Day 1:** 99 g (about 3½ ounces or ½ cup cooked); about 1 ounce (28 g) uncooked; note that this can vary with different types of pasta

+ **Day 2:** break day

+ **Day 3:** 148 g (about 5 ounces or ⅔ cup cooked); about 1.6 ounces (45 g) uncooked

+ **Day 4:** break day

+ **Day 5:** 222 g (about 8 ounces or 1 cup cooked); 2 ounces (56 g) uncooked

+ **Day 6:** break day

WHITE BREAD:

+ **Day 1:** 26 g, about 1 slice

+ **Day 2:** break day

+ **Day 3:** 39 g, about 1½ slices

+ **Day 4:** break day

+ **Day 5:** 52 g, about 2 slices

+ **Day 6:** break day

The low-FODMAP diet is *not* a gluten-free diet. FODMAPs are carbohydrates while gluten is a protein. Symptoms that arise from eating wheat-containing products may be related to the fructans in the wheat, and not the gluten.

SPAGHETTI AGLIO E OLIO

This is a classic Italian recipe for spaghetti aglio e olio. Spaghetti aglio e olio originated in Naples and uses the staples of pasta, olive oil, garlic, parsley, and Parmigiano-Reggiano cheese. I incorporate a little extra color and flavor by adding kale and use a garlic-infused oil to keep this recipe low FODMAP. You are going to have so much fun enjoying this impressive meal.

Bring a pot of salted water to a boil and cook the pasta according to the package directions until al dente. Reserve ½ cup (120 ml) of the pasta cooking water before draining the pasta.

Heat the infused oil in a large skillet over medium heat. Add the red pepper flakes, then the kale, salt, and several grinds of pepper. Cook until the kale is wilted, up to 1 minute, tossing occasionally. Add the drained spaghetti and toss to coat in the oil. Stir in the lemon zest and juice. Add some of the reserved pasta water, 1 tablespoon (15 ml) at a time, until it is your desired consistency. Garnish with the parsley and serve topped with the pine nuts and Parmesan, if using.

VARIATION: Use low-FODMAP, gluten-free pasta to enjoy this during the FODMAP elimination phase.

TIP: Freshly grated Parmesan cheese tastes completely different from the powdered stuff you buy in canisters at the supermarket. For best results, do not substitute pre-grated Parmesan in this recipe.

NOTE: For the first days of the challenge, you may consume less than a typical serving size for this meal; for the last day, it may be slightly more. See "Portion Size vs. Serving Size," page 29.

6 ounces (170 g) *uncooked* spaghetti (will yield about 3 cups cooked); adjust personal portion based on day of challenge:

+ **Day 1: 99 g (3½ ounces or about ½ cup)** *cooked*

+ **Day 3: 148 g (5 ounces or about ⅔ cup)** *cooked*

+ **Day 5: 222 g (8 ounces or about 1 cup)** *cooked*

¼ cup (60 ml) garlic-infused oil

¼ teaspoon red pepper flakes

1 large bunch kale, about 5 stalks, stemmed and chopped

½ teaspoon salt

Freshly ground black pepper

1 teaspoon lemon zest

1 teaspoon lemon juice

2 tablespoons (8 g) chopped fresh parsley

3 tablespoons (27 g) toasted pine nuts (see Note, page 48)

Freshly grated Parmesan, for serving (omit for vegan or dairy-free version)

* **Nutritional analysis for this recipe is calculated based on the standard serving size,** *not* **the recommended portion for FODMAP reintroduction testing.**

NUTRITION PER SERVING*: Serving Size: 137 g, Calories: 320, Total Fat: 19 g, Saturated Fat: 2.5 g, Carbohydrates: 32 g, Sugar: 1 g, Sodium: 430 mg, Fiber: 3 g, Protein: 7 g

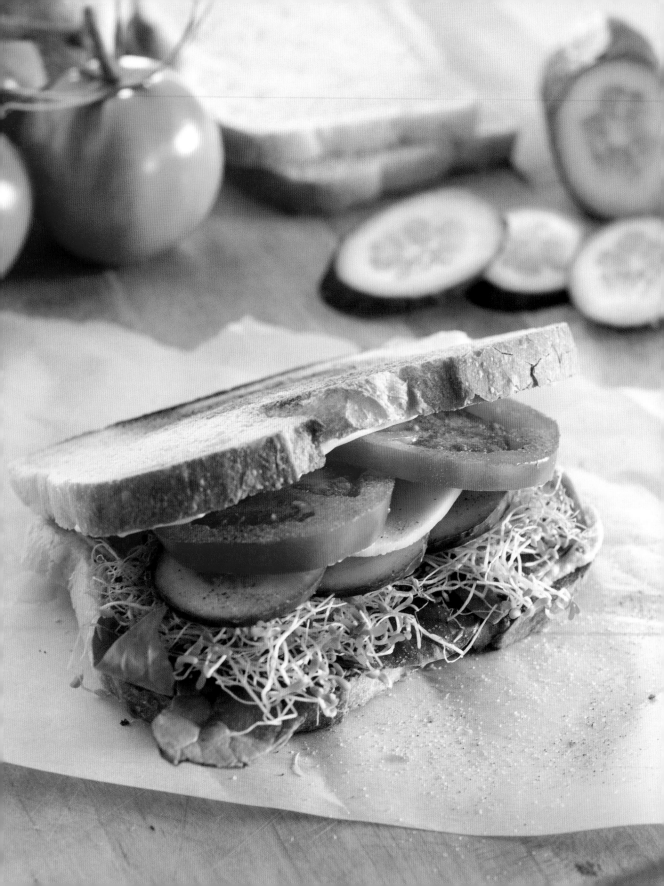

HEARTY VEGETABLE SANDWICH

I love a hearty sandwich filled with vegetables, savory spreads, and cheese. This sandwich piles the veggies on so high you may have trouble biting into it. You can use tahini (sesame seed paste) or hummus for this recipe; just note that commercially bought hummus will not be low FODMAP. See my blog at www.rachelpaulsfood.com for a great hummus recipe that uses canned chickpeas.

Lightly toast the bread and spread one side with tahini or hummus and the other with mayonnaise. Divide the sandwich ingredients between two of the slices and season lightly with salt and pepper. Fold sides together and slice as desired.

*Select a mayonnaise with low-FODMAP ingredients (no added onion and garlic), such as Hellmann's.

VARIATION: To enjoy this on the FODMAP elimination phase, use only low-FODMAP bread.

2 slices bread, white bread and low-FODMAP bread combination; adjust portion based on day of challenge:

+ **Day 1: 26 g, about 1 slice white bread, 1 slice low-FODMAP bread**

+ **Day 3: 39 g, about 1½ slices white bread, ½ slice low-FODMAP bread**

+ **Day 5: 56 g, about 2 slices white bread, no low-FODMAP bread**

2 teaspoons tahini or low-FODMAP hummus

1 teaspoon mayonnaise*

1 slice (20 g) provolone cheese (omit for vegan or dairy-free version)

3 (10 g) spinach leaves

3 or 4 slices common cucumber

¼ cup (5 g) alfalfa sprouts

2 ripe tomato slices

Salt and pepper to taste

NUTRITION PER SERVING (DAY 1): Serving Size: 159 g, Calories: 330, Total Fat: 16 g, Saturated Fat: 5 g, Carbohydrates: 38 g, Sugar: 5 g, Sodium: 460 mg, Fiber: 1 g, Protein: 11 g

FRUCTANS: ONION

We are now at the onion challenge. Because onions are such a common IBS trigger, this challenge may seem a bit scary. I can understand that sentiment. Although I loved onions for the majority of my life, I have learned they are bothersome for my body unless in very small amounts.

While I hope your results are different from mine, it is not a failure if you have a negative reaction. You will be better off having the knowledge to move forward! If you react to a certain amount of onion, then stop the challenge and shift to a break period. Feel reassured that you can still enjoy so many foods and flavors. Don't let this discourage you from continuing with the reintroduction process.

You can use any type of onion for this challenge, just make sure to weigh your onion raw using the recommended portion sizes on the right.

ONION:

+ **Day 1: 11 g raw onion**

+ **Day 2: break day**

+ **Day 3: 22 g raw onion**

+ **Day 4: break day**

+ **Day 5: 44 g raw onion**

+ **Day 6: break day**

I personally much prefer the flavor of cooked onion to raw. Check out my amazing recipes to follow.

WHAT TO DO IF SYMPTOMS BEGIN
If you start to experience symptoms with a challenge, just stop the challenge and move on to the break period. This does not mean that you are doomed never to enjoy that food category again. You can opt to repeat the challenge later, possibly starting with a smaller amount of the challenge food.

FRENCH ONION BAKED POTATO

Here is my short and sweet recipe inspired by baked "French onion" soup. If you've been missing that flavor profile, you will love this baked potato. To enjoy this on the FODMAP elimination phase, omit the onion altogether and enjoy this as a cheesy stuffed potato instead!

Place the onion in a microwave-safe dish and cover with plastic wrap, cutting a small slit in the plastic. Cook on high for 2 to 3 minutes, then remove and drain the water from the dish. Stir in the butter and pinch of sugar and return to the microwave, covering again with the wrap for another 30 seconds to 1 minute. The onion will shrink with cooking. Remove and set aside.

Line a plate with paper towels. Pierce the potato with a fork and arrange it on the prepared plate. Microwave on high for 6 to 10 minutes, depending on your microwave, until done. Cut the potato in half lengthwise and scoop out the pulp, leaving a ¼-inch (6 mm) thick shell on both halves. Combine the potato pulp, half of the cooked onions, 2 tablespoons (10 g) of the cheese, sour cream, salt, and pepper in a small bowl and mash together. Add the milk as needed to smooth the consistency. Spoon the potato mixture evenly into each shell and top with remaining onions and cheese. Microwave again for 30 seconds to 1 minute until the cheese is melted.

NOTE: Using the microwave to cook the potato and onion makes the recipe a cinch, and perfect for hot days.

Red onion, thinly sliced; adjust portion based on day of challenge:

+ **Day 1: 11 g raw onion**

+ **Day 3: 22 g raw onion**

+ **Day 5: 44 g raw onion**

1 teaspoon butter

Pinch of sugar

1 (170 g) medium baking potato

4 tablespoons (20 g) shredded Gruyère cheese, divided

1 tablespoon (15 g) lactose-free sour cream

¼ teaspoon salt

⅛ teaspoon freshly ground black pepper

1 to 2 teaspoons low-FODMAP milk, such as lactose-free or almond milk

NUTRITION PER SERVING (DAY 1): Serving Size: 228 g, Calories: 320, Total Fat: 17 g, Saturated Fat: 11 g, Carbohydrates: 33 g, Sugar: 3 g, Sodium: 780 mg, Fiber: 2 g, Protein: 11 g

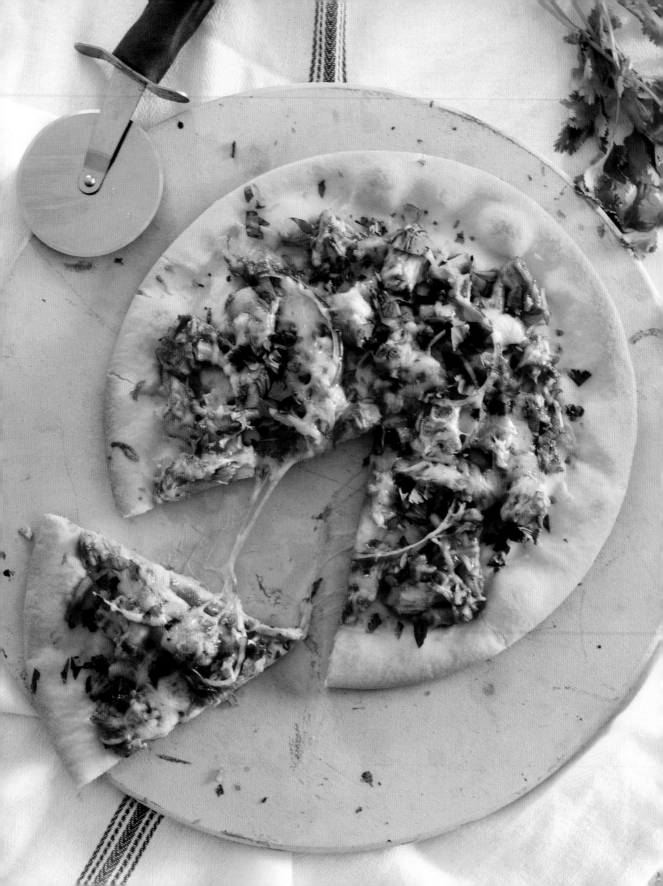

HOMEMADE BBQ CHICKEN PIZZA

When I lived in St. Louis for my residency, one of my favorite places to eat was California Pizza Kitchen. I would always order the Barbecue Chicken Pizza. It's even better homemade—absolutely irresistible.

Preheat the oven based on the recommended setting for your selected pizza crust. Brush the crust lightly with the oil. In a medium bowl, toss the chicken with the barbecue sauce and then spread the chicken and sauce over the crust. Layer the cheeses and onion on top of the chicken. Transfer the pizza to the oven and bake for 7 to 10 minutes (or according to your brand's recommendations). Remove from the oven and top with fresh cilantro, if desired. Slice the pizza and serve immediately.

VARIATION: Omit the onion to enjoy this on the FODMAP elimination phase.

TIP: Commercial barbecue sauce may be low FODMAP in servings up to 2 tablespoons (30 ml). However, if you are uncertain, there are low-FODMAP-certified products that are available. I also have a recipe for low-FODMAP barbecue sauce at www.rachelpaulsfood.com.

NOTE: I like UDI's gluten-free individual pizza crusts and Schär's pizza crusts for easy options.

1 (4-ounce [114 g]) low-FODMAP, gluten-free personal pizza crust

1 teaspoon olive oil or garlic-infused olive oil

2 ounces (56 g) chopped or shredded cooked chicken (see Tip, page 53)

2 tablespoons (30 ml) low-FODMAP barbecue sauce, gluten-free if necessary (see Tip)

3 tablespoons (15 g) shredded mozzarella

2 tablespoons (15 g) shredded smoked Gouda cheese

Red onion, thinly sliced; adjust portion based on day of challenge:

+ **Day 1: 11 g raw onion**

+ **Day 3: 22 g raw onion**

+ **Day 5: 44 g raw onion**

Chopped fresh cilantro, for topping (optional)

NUTRITION PER SERVING (DAY 1): Serving Size: 247 g, Calories: 630, Total Fat: 23 g, Saturated Fat: 5 g, Carbohydrates: 73 g, Sugar: 13 g, Sodium: 1360 mg, Fiber: 3 g, Protein: 31 g

FRUCTANS: GARLIC

Vampires beware! You are going to be trying garlic now.

This challenge will involve introducing very small amounts of garlic. You won't even start with a full clove. By the end of the challenge, if you tolerate 4 grams you will have "passed."

Tolerating this challenge will allow you to enjoy several garlic-containing foods. However, don't assume you can consume the garlic bread or Caesar salad at your favorite restaurant. Amounts of garlic in some recipes could be much more than 4 grams, so be cautious in your selections.

I recommend using a scale to weigh the garlic, as there is a variation in the size of cloves in each head. The recommended portion sizes are in the list on the right.

GARLIC:

+ **Day 1: 1 g, about ½ clove garlic**

+ **Day 2: break day**

+ **Day 3: 2 g, about 1 clove garlic**

+ **Day 4: break day**

+ **Day 5: 4 g, about 2 cloves garlic**

+ **Day 6: break day**

You can eat the garlic raw or cooked, but I personally much prefer the flavor of cooked garlic. See the following recipes for some ideas.

Garlic may be high in FODMAPs, but if you plant a garlic head in soil and place it in some sunlight, in just a few weeks, little curly green plants will grow. These stalks, or shoots, are also known as garlic scapes. Garlic shoots are lower in FODMAPs than garlic cloves (Monash lists a low-FODMAP serving at 30 grams).

Although the shoots have a flavor slightly less potent than garlic, they can be a delicious substitute for the real thing. A great idea to pursue after this challenge if you still find garlic troublesome for your tummy!

WHOLE ROASTED GARLIC CLOVES

In my pre-IBS days I would often roast an entire garlic head, then mash it up and spread on crusty bread for my husband and me to share. The roasting process caramelizes the garlic and makes it taste incredible.

Preheat the oven or toaster oven to 400°F (200°C, or gas mark 6). Slice the top of the garlic head off and place the entire head on a piece of aluminum foil. Drizzle the oil over the head and rub it in, then wrap the head in the foil to completely encase it. Place the foil-wrapped head on a small baking sheet and bake for about 30 minutes, until the cloves are soft. To remove each clove, gently apply pressure to the base of the head and it will slide right out.

NOTE: Enjoy these roasted cloves spread on a low-FODMAP cracker or piece of bread, or sprinkle them over your favorite dish.

1 head garlic; adjust portion based on day of challenge:

+ **Day 1: 1 g, about ½ clove garlic**

+ **Day 3: 2 g, about 1 clove garlic**

+ **Day 5: 4 g, about 2 cloves garlic**

1 teaspoon olive oil

NUTRITION PER SERVING*: Serving Size: 1.7 g,
Calories: 10, Total Fat: 1 g, Saturated Fat: 0 g, Carbohydrates: 0 g,
Sugar: 0 g, Sodium: 0 mg, Fiber: 0 g, Protein: 0 g

* Nutritional analysis for this recipe is calculated based on the standard serving size, *not* the recommended portion for FODMAP reintroduction testing.

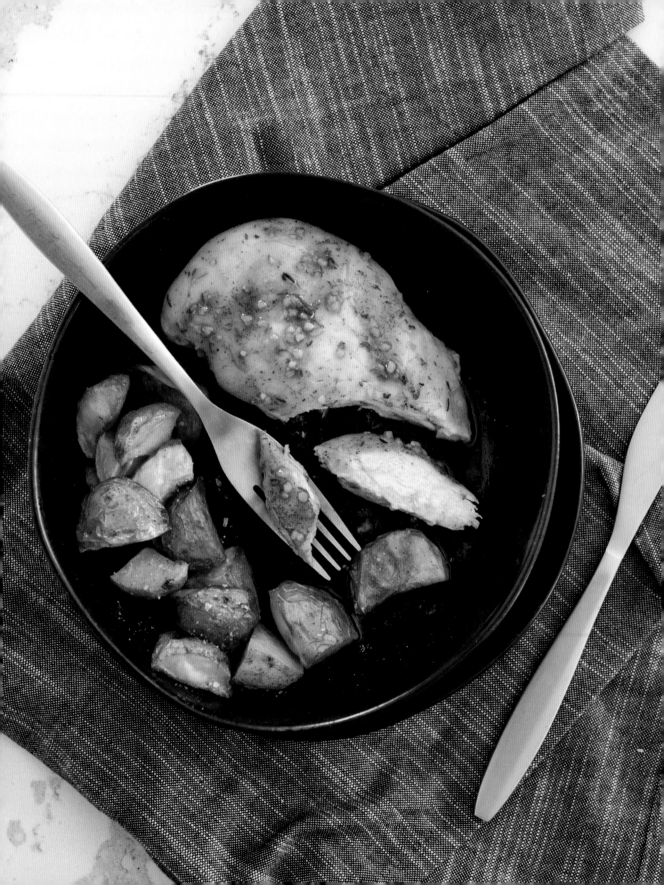

MAPLE MUSTARD CHICKEN FOR ONE

This maple mustard chicken is a simple, easy, and delectable dinner for one. It is great with or without the garlic. My personal favorite for a busy weeknight.

Preheat the oven or toaster oven to 400°F (200°C, or gas mark 6). Spray a small baking dish with nonstick cooking spray.

Combine the mustard, maple syrup, lemon juice, thyme, and garlic in a small bowl and set aside. Lay the chicken between two pieces of parchment paper or plastic wrap and beat with a mallet until ½ inch (1.3 cm) thick. Season liberally with salt and pepper. Place the chicken in the prepared baking dish, then pour the sauce evenly on top of the chicken. Cover with foil and bake for 20 minutes, or until the chicken is cooked through (internal temperature 165°F [73°C]). Serve immediately.

NOTE: This recipe easily doubles or triples; just be aware that the baking time may increase with added chicken.

1 tablespoon (15 g) Dijon mustard

1 tablespoon (15 ml) maple syrup

1 teaspoon lemon juice

⅛ teaspoon thyme

Garlic, finely minced; adjust portion based on day of challenge:

+ **Day 1: 1 g, about ½ clove garlic**

+ **Day 3: 2 g, about 1 clove garlic**

+ **Day 5: 4 g, about 2 cloves garlic**

6 ounces (168 g) boneless, skinless chicken breast

Salt and pepper to taste

NUTRITION PER SERVING (DAY 1): Serving Size: 209 g, Calories: 270, Total Fat: 4.5 g, Saturated Fat: 1 g, Carbohydrates: 14 g, Sugar: 12 g, Sodium: 440 mg, Fiber: 0 g, Protein: 38 g

GALACTANS (GOS)

We have reached the final FODMAP category: galactans, or GOS, which is short for galacto-oligosaccharides. These are chains of galactose sugars joined together with a glucose molecule at the end. There is no human enzyme capable of breaking down the bonds between the galactose sugars, so they move through the gut unabsorbed. An excess intake may lead to gas, bloating, and GI upset, as well as potential symptom flares in people with IBS.

On the positive side, these prebiotic FODMAPs are a common energy source for gut bacteria and help them thrive. Therefore, finding out whether you tolerate GOS can enhance your intestinal microbiome (see "The Intestinal Microbiome," page 23) and overall health.

The recommended test foods for GOS are almonds and canned chickpeas/garbanzo beans. Feel free to enjoy these foods as they are. Munch on a bag of salted almonds, throw the chickpeas into your salad, or try one of the recipes detailed in this section. To keep your gut happy, stick to my suggested testing portions, and be sure to keep track of the results in your journal.

The recommended portion sizes for using almonds or chickpeas/garbanzo beans to test GOS are in the list on the right.

ALMONDS:

+ Day 1: 18 g, about 15 nuts
+ Day 2: break day
+ Day 3: 24 g, about 20 nuts
+ Day 4: break day
+ Day 5: 36 g, about 30 nuts
+ Day 6: break day

CANNED CHICKPEAS/GARBANZO BEANS, DRAINED AND RINSED:

+ Day 1: 84 g, about ½ cup
+ Day 2: break day
+ Day 3: 112 g, about ⅔ cup
+ Day 4: break day
+ Day 5: 168 g, about 1 cup
+ Day 6: break day

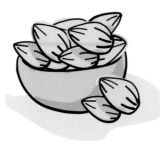

CANDIED ALMONDS

These are one of my go-to snacks. Dangerously addictive, these cinnamon sugar almonds remind me of the nuts sold by roaster carts all over Manhattan. Use these in place of the almonds on my Orange Almond Salad (page 127) to make it extra fabulous.

Preheat the oven to 250°F (120°C, or gas mark ½) and place a rack in the center of the oven. Grease a large baking sheet with baking spray.

In a small bowl, combine the sugar, salt, and cinnamon. Set aside.

In a large mixing bowl, whip the egg white and vanilla with a whisk until frothy, about 1 minute. Toss the almonds in the egg whites until coated, then sprinkle the sugar/spice mixture over the almonds. Mix to combine well. Spread the almonds in a single layer on the prepared baking sheet. Transfer the sheet to the oven and bake for approximately 1 hour, stirring the almonds and rotating the tray every 15 minutes to ensure even cooking, until slightly browned and aromatic. Remove the tray from the oven and let the almonds cool on the tray before serving. You can enjoy them warm or at room temperature. Store in an airtight container at room temperature, or freeze.

VARIATION: You can make any nuts taste better with this recipe. Try peanuts, pecans, or walnuts to enjoy this snack during the FODMAP elimination phase.

NOTE: These are delicious on top of vanilla ice cream, stirred into yogurt, or on their own as a crunchy treat.

¾ cup (150 g) sugar

1 teaspoon salt

2 teaspoons ground cinnamon

1 egg white

1 tablespoon (15 ml) vanilla extract

1 pound (450 g) raw whole almonds; adjust personal portion based on day of challenge:

+ **Day 1: 18 g, about 15 nuts**

+ **Day 3: 24 g, about 20 nuts**

+ **Day 5: 36 g, about 30 nuts**

NUTRITION PER SERVING*: Serving Size: 27 g, Calories: 130, Total Fat: 9 g, Saturated Fat: 0.5 g, Carbohydrates: 10 g, Sugar: 7 g, Sodium: 100 mg, Fiber: 3 g, Protein: 4 g

* Nutritional analysis for this recipe is calculated based on the standard serving size, *not* the recommended portion for FODMAP reintroduction testing.

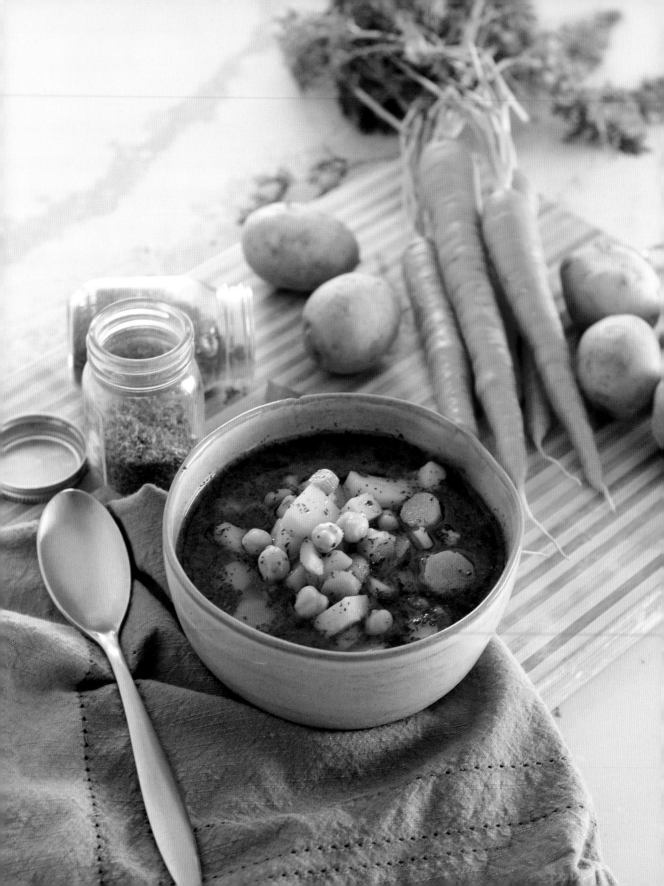

CHICKPEA AND POTATO SOUP

This nourishing vegan soup uses canned chickpeas (garbanzo beans) for added flavor, texture, and fiber. For non-vegans, you can substitute a low-FODMAP chicken soup base and add some precooked chicken to the broth as well. Super satisfying.

In a saucepan, warm the olive oil over medium heat. Add the potatoes, carrots, and parsnips and sauté for about 5 minutes until the carrots and parsnips have softened slightly. Stir in the broth, bay leaf, basil, thyme, and paprika. Bring to a boil, then lower the heat to medium-low. Cover and simmer until the vegetables are tender but not mushy, 20 to 30 minutes. Add the infused oil, then taste the broth and add salt and pepper as desired. Stir the chickpeas into each portion prior to serving. Serve hot.

TIP: I recommend Yukon gold or other yellow potato for this soup. They are a low- to medium-starch potato and work well with recipes that involve roasting, mashing, soups, and chowders.

1 tablespoon (15 ml) olive oil

2 cups (220 g) peeled and chopped Yukon gold potatoes

3 medium carrots (200 g), peeled and chopped

3 parsnips (130 g), peeled and chopped

3 cups (705 ml) low-FODMAP vegetable broth or stock, gluten-free if necessary (see Note, page 61)

1 bay leaf

1 teaspoon dried basil

½ teaspoon dried thyme

¼ teaspoon paprika

1 tablespoon (15 ml) garlic-infused oil

Salt and pepper to taste

1 (15-ounce [420 g]) can chickpeas, drained and rinsed; adjust personal portion based on day of challenge:

+ **Day 1: 84 g, about ½ cup**

+ **Day 3: 112 g, about ⅔ cup**

+ **Day 5: 168 g, about 1 cup**

NUTRITION PER SERVING*: Serving Size: 290 g, Calories: 220, Total Fat: 7 g, Saturated Fat: 1 g, Carbohydrates: 34 g, Sugar: 7 g, Sodium: 540 mg, Fiber: 8 g, Protein: 7 g

* Nutritional analysis for this recipe is calculated based on the standard serving size, *not* the recommended portion for FODMAP reintroduction testing.

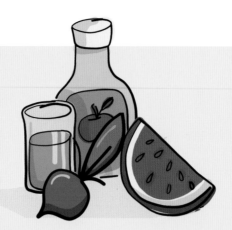

REINTRODUCTION, STAGE 3
FODMAP COMBINATION FOODS

Congratulations! You have made it through the first two stages of reintroduction and are well on your way to figuring out which FODMAPs you can add back to your diet! I am so proud of you. I bet you can't believe you have made it this far.

Now is the exciting *combination* phase of reintroduction. The combination foods in this phase will incorporate two FODMAP categories that you have *successfully tolerated* earlier. Testing more than one FODMAP at a time brings you closer to the final phase of the low-FODMAP lifestyle: integration and personalization.

Of course, like the earlier tests, challenges are optional if you don't intend to combine these FODMAP subgroups as part of your usual diet. You can opt to test the foods that you are most comfortable with or most interested in consuming. If you need a break, then feel free to pause at this point. You have certainly earned it!

For this stage, you can test three days in a row, or continue testing a day at a time with the break days in between. There are no strict rules, so follow the pattern that fits your digestive system and your schedule. I tend to be on the conservative side, so I prefer to schedule a break day between test days, particularly when incorporating fructans and GOS into the challenges as discussed below.

The Monash app specifically outlines only two combination challenges. These are sorbitol with fructose and GOS with fructans. However, I will provide you choices for other combinations that you may wish to test. There will be fewer options and recipes for these challenges because they are not as well delineated.

COMBINATION CHALLENGE

SORBITOL AND FRUCTOSE

Your first combination challenge will test sorbitol and fructose. The recommended test foods for this challenge are Pink Lady apples and cherries. If you choose to test using apples, make sure they are Pink Ladies. Other apple varieties may contain higher levels or different subgroups of FODMAPs; do not substitute.

These fruit choices are lovely on their own, stirred into yogurt, or tossed in a salad or smoothie. I enjoy slices of apples with a dollop of peanut butter or nestled in a grilled cheese sandwich. You can also fold an apple wedge and cube of Gouda cheese into a slice of deli turkey for a low-carb snack.

The correct portion sizes for testing Pink Lady apples and cherries are in the list on the right.

PINK LADY APPLES:

+ **Day 1: 42 g, about ¼ medium**
+ **Day 2: 83 g, about ½ medium**
+ **Day 3: 166 g, about 1 medium**

CHERRIES:

+ **Day 1: 28 g, about 5 cherries**
+ **Day 2: 56 g, about 8 cherries**
+ **Day 3: 70 g, about 10 cherries**

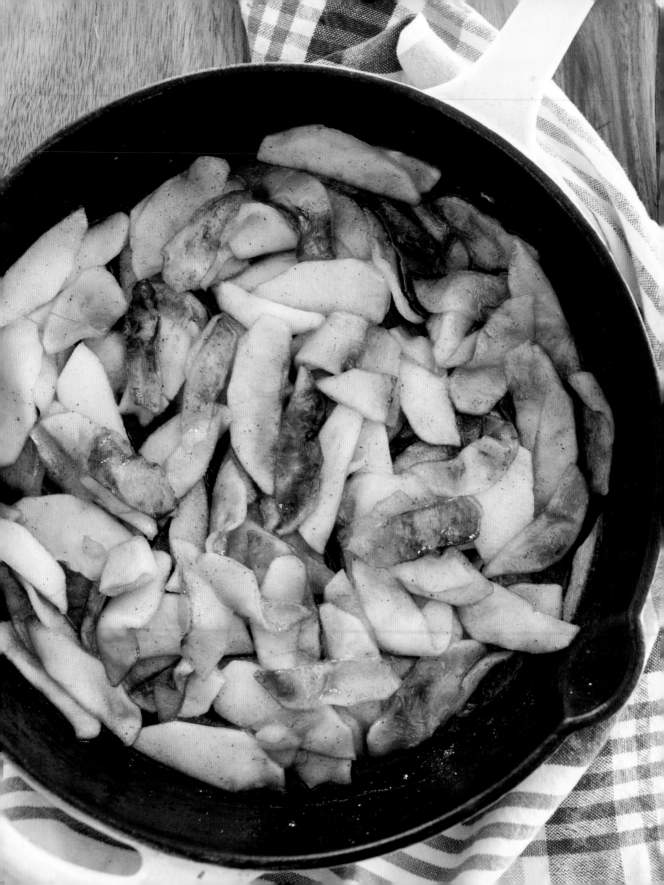

FRIED APPLES

Fried apples are a sweet treat that hail from our Southern states. They are amazing plain or as a topping for oatmeal, ice cream, yogurt, waffles, and pancakes.

Peel, core, and chop the apples into ¼-inch (6 mm) slices, then weigh out 166 g for cooking. Rub the lemon juice over the apple slices to prevent browning. In a 9-inch (23 cm) cast-iron skillet over medium-low heat, melt the butter. Stir in the brown sugar, salt, cinnamon, and vanilla and cook for about 20 seconds. Increase the heat to medium, then add the apple slices and stir to coat with the sugar. Cook, stirring occasionally, for 10 to 15 minutes until the slices are soft. Serve warm.

TIP: Squeezing lemon juice over apple slices keeps them from turning brown in color, a great trick to keep any fruit platter looking its best.

3 medium Pink Lady apples; adjust personal portion based on day of challenge:

+ **Day 1: 42 g, about ¼ medium apple**

+ **Day 2: 83 g, about ½ medium apple**

+ **Day 3: 166 g, about 1 medium apple**

½ teaspoon lemon juice

1½ tablespoons (23 g) unsalted butter

1 tablespoon (12 g) packed dark brown sugar

Pinch of salt

¼ teaspoon ground cinnamon

¼ teaspoon vanilla extract

NUTRITION PER SERVING*: Serving Size: 103 g, Calories: 150, Total Fat: 9 g, Saturated Fat: 6 g, Carbohydrates: 18 g, Sugar: 15 g, Sodium: 75 mg, Fiber: 2 g, Protein: 0 g

* Nutritional analysis for this recipe is calculated based on the standard serving size, *not* the recommended portion for FODMAP reintroduction testing.

GOS AND FRUCTANS

Your second combination challenge is GOS and fructans. Because this challenge incorporates the more complex fructans, I recommend using the challenge schedule that alternates test days with break days.

The recommended test foods for this combination challenge are pearl barley, cashews, and whole-grain wheat bread. You can enjoy them on their own or incorporate them into another recipe. My Candied Almonds recipe (page 147) works great for the cashews, and my Hearty Vegetable Sandwich recipe (page 137) is superb for the whole-grain wheat bread.

I have also included a recipe for cooking pearl barley. I love using pearl barley as a salad topper or mixed into my favorite soup. You can also serve it as a side dish or breakfast choice.

Note that both pearl barley and wheat bread contain gluten, so if you are sensitive or intolerant, I recommend avoiding these for your challenge foods.

The correct portion sizes for testing pearl barley, cashews, and whole-grain wheat bread are listed on the right.

PEARL BARLEY (COOKED WEIGHT):

+ **Day 1: 56 g, about ¼ cup**

+ **Day 2: break day**

+ **Day 3: 112 g, about ½ cup**

+ **Day 4: break day**

+ **Day 5: 224 g, about 1 cup**

CASHEWS:

+ **Day 1: 15 g, about 10 nuts**

+ **Day 2: break day**

+ **Day 3: 30 g, about 20 nuts**

+ **Day 4: break day**

+ **Day 5: 45 g, about 30 nuts**

BREAD, WHOLE-GRAIN WHEAT:

+ **Day 1: 36 g, about 1½ slices**

+ **Day 2: break day**

+ **Day 3: 48 g, about 2 slices**

+ **Day 4: break day**

+ **Day 5: 72 g, about 3 slices**

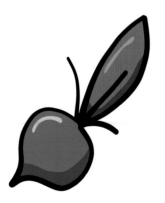

COOKED PEARL BARLEY

Pearl barley is a starchy grain that is excellent for making soups. It is low in fat and high in fiber and essential nutrients.

Add the barley, broth, and salt to a large pot. Cover and bring to a boil over medium-high heat. Decrease the heat to a low simmer and continue cooking, covered, for 25 to 30 minutes, until the barley is soft and has absorbed most of the liquid. There may be some excess liquid that you can drain off if desired. Remove from the heat and allow it to rest, covered, for 10 minutes, then stir in the olive oil. Fluff with a fork and serve. May be stored in the refrigerator for 3 to 5 days, or freezer for up to 1 month.

NOTE: Make a pearl barley "bowl" by adding low-FODMAP servings of sliced carrots, common cucumber, tomato, cooked chicken, and avocado. Drizzle with a little balsamic vinegar and olive oil and enjoy!

¾ cup (135 g) *uncooked* pearl barley, rinsed and drained; adjust personal portion based on day of challenge:

+ **Day 1: 56 g, about ¼ cup** *cooked*

+ **Day 3: 112 g, about ½ cup** *cooked*

+ **Day 5: 224 g, about 1 cup** *cooked*

2½ cups (590 ml) low-FODMAP vegetable broth or stock, gluten-free if necessary (see Note, page 61)

½ teaspoon salt (optional, depending on how salty your broth is)

1 teaspoon olive oil

NUTRITION PER SERVING*: Serving Size: 230 g, Calories: 180, Total Fat: 2 g, Saturated Fat: 0 g, Carbohydrates: 37 g, Sugar: 1 g, Sodium: 550 mg, Fiber: 7 g, Protein: 5 g

* Nutritional analysis for this recipe is calculated based on the standard serving size, *not* **the recommended portion for FODMAP reintroduction testing.**

FRUCTANS AND FRUCTOSE

Your third combination challenge is fructans and fructose. Once again, because this challenge contains fructans, I suggest incorporating break days between your test days.

For this challenge the recommended test food is Jerusalem artichokes. Jerusalem artichokes, or sunchokes, are root vegetables that are completely different from regular artichokes. They are full of the prebiotic inulin fructan. To test this food, I highly recommend using my Jerusalem Artichokes with Balsamic and Rosemary Browned Butter recipe (page 157). I absolutely adore this recipe. It's a gourmet treat that everyone will swoon over.

The recommended portion sizes for testing Jerusalem artichokes are noted on the right. Please note that this challenge is not formally outlined in the Monash app. Therefore, the amounts of food suggested are based on my recommendations and other expert opinions.

JERUSALEM ARTICHOKES:

+ **Day 1: 30 g**

+ **Day 2: break day**

+ **Day 3: 65 g**

+ **Day 4: break day**

+ **Day 5: 100 g**

Jerusalem artichokes are more popular in Europe than in America and, similar to ginger roots, have light brown skin. They are approximately 3 to 4 inches (7.6 to 10 cm) long and 1 to 2 inches (2.5 to 5 cm) wide. Although they can be eaten raw, you may prefer them steamed, baked, fried, or boiled (similar to a potato). In North America, the season for sunchokes is typically October through April, but they are usually available year-round. If you can't find them at your local store, check out specialty groceries or Amazon.

JERUSALEM ARTICHOKES WITH BALSAMIC AND ROSEMARY BROWNED BUTTER

I love the flavor of browned butter, but infusing it with rosemary makes it even better. You can improve any vegetable with this deluxe dressing.

Heat the oil in a heavy skillet with a lid over medium-high (see Tip). Add the Jerusalem artichokes and water to the skillet and season with salt and pepper. Cover and cook, stirring occasionally, until the artichokes are tender, about 8 minutes. Uncover the skillet and drain the water, then return the skillet to the heat and continue cooking until the artichokes are crisp and brown, about 10 minutes. Transfer to a platter to keep warm.

Add the rosemary and butter to the skillet and cook, stirring often, until the butter foams, then browns, about 4 minutes. It will have a slight nutty aroma. Watch carefully so it doesn't burn. Remove the skillet from the heat quickly and pour the browned butter into a serving bowl. Remove the rosemary sprigs and stir in the balsamic vinegar. Serve the artichokes drizzled with the browned butter.

VARIATION: Asparagus is an amazing substitution in this recipe! No need to chop the spears. Plan 5 minutes for the first step (cooking until tender), and 2 to 3 minutes for crisping. The rest of the recipe is unchanged.

TIP: I prefer to use a white-bottomed saucepan or skillet when browning butter, so you can see the point when the brown flecks form. This will help you avoid burning it.

1 tablespoon (15 ml) olive oil

1 pound (455 g) Jerusalem artichokes (about 4 to 5), scrubbed and quartered; adjust personal portion based on day of challenge:

+ **Day 1: 30 g**

+ **Day 3: 65 g**

+ **Day 5: 100 g**

5 tablespoons (75 ml) water

Kosher salt and freshly ground black pepper

2 sprigs rosemary

¼ cup (60 g) unsalted butter

3 tablespoons (45 ml) balsamic vinegar

* Nutritional analysis for this recipe is calculated based on the standard serving size, *not* the recommended portion for FODMAP reintroduction testing.

NUTRITION PER SERVING*: Serving Size: 82 g, Calories: 120, Total Fat: 8 g, Saturated Fat: 4 g, Carbohydrates: 11 g, Sugar: 6 g, Sodium: 0 mg, Fiber: 1 g, Protein: 1 g

SORBITOL AND FRUCTANS

Your final combination challenge—and the final challenge in this book!—is sorbitol and fructans. This is a common FODMAP combination found in stone fruits. If you have missed plums in your menu, here is the opportunity to see whether you tolerate them.

The recommended test food for this challenge is Black Diamond plums. You can eat these on their own or use my quick and delicious Five-Minute Microwave Plum Crisp recipe (page 159). Feel free to test this food three days in a row, or with break days in between.

The recommended portion sizes for testing Black Diamond plums are noted on the right. As with the previous challenge, this FODMAP combination is not formally outlined in the Monash app. Therefore, the amounts of food suggested are based on my recommendations and other expert opinions.

BLACK DIAMOND PLUMS:

+ **Day 1: 30 g, about ½ plum**

+ **Day 2: break day**

+ **Day 3: 66 g, about 1 plum**

+ **Day 4: break day**

+ **Day 5: 100 g, about 1½ plums**

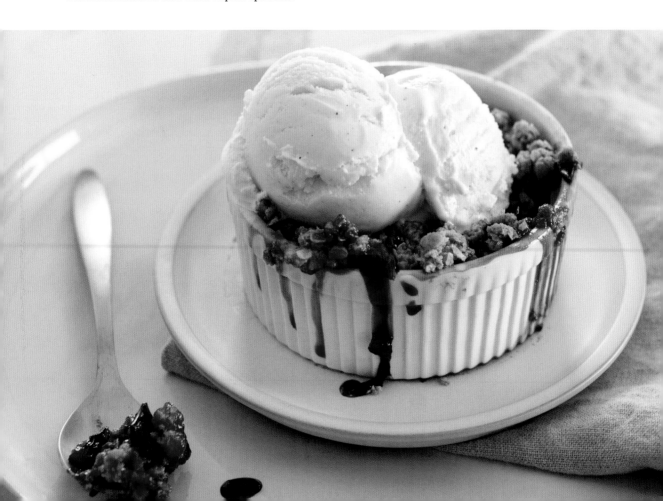

FIVE-MINUTE MICROWAVE PLUM CRISP

This single-serving recipe for a microwaved fruit crisp is the perfect way to satisfy your craving for baked goods without warming up the oven. It tastes fantastic topped with low-FODMAP ice cream. FODMAP fact: FODMAPs are not detected in rhubarb, so you can enjoy this fruit at whim.

Mix the fruit, granulated sugar, cornstarch, and vanilla together in a medium shallow ramekin or microwave-safe dish. This is the bottom layer of your crisp. In a separate small bowl, mix the coconut oil, quick-cooking oats, light brown sugar, cinnamon, and flour by hand to form a chunky dough. Sprinkle the oat mixture on top of the fruit in the microwave-safe dish. Microwave for 2 to 3 minutes until the fruit starts to bubble (microwave ovens will vary). Allow to sit for 3 to 5 minutes to cool, then enjoy warm.

VARIATION: This recipe is easily modifiable to use only rhubarb, or a rhubarb-berry (strawberry, raspberry, or blueberry) combination. Just check your portion size to ensure you are sticking to a low-FODMAP amount to enjoy during the FODMAP elimination phase.

TIP: If your fruit is very tart, you may wish to increase the sugar in the bottom layer.

Fruit, total amount of 100 g; adjust portion based on the day of the challenge:

+ **Day 1: 30 g plum, cubed or diced, and 70 g rhubarb (fresh or frozen, defrosted), chopped**

+ **Day 3: 66 g plum, cubed or diced, and 34 g rhubarb, chopped**

+ **Day 5: 100 g plum, cubed or diced**

2 teaspoons granulated sugar

1¼ teaspoons cornstarch

½ teaspoon vanilla extract

1½ tablespoons (23 ml) melted coconut oil

2 tablespoons plus 2 teaspoons (13 g) quick-cooking oats

1½ tablespoons (18 g) packed light brown sugar

½ teaspoon ground cinnamon

2 tablespoons (16 g) low-FODMAP, gluten-free flour

NUTRITION PER SERVING (DAY 1): Serving Size: 183 g, Calories: 440, Total Fat: 22 g, Saturated Fat: 18 g, Carbohydrates: 59 g, Sugar: 31 g, Sodium: 10 mg, Fiber: 4 g, Protein: 3 g

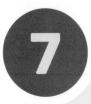

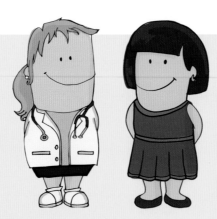

INTEGRATION AND PERSONALIZATION:

THE FINAL LOW-FODMAP PHASE

Congratulations! You have officially completed the structured challenges of the reintroduction phase. Now is the start of the final phase of the low-FODMAP diet: integration and personalization. In this phase, you will begin to gradually expand your menu, using the knowledge that you have gained so far.

Phase 3 is a much less formal, individually driven phase than the previous two, and the information in this chapter will reflect that. The point of integration and personalization is to fine-tune your understanding of your personal tolerances, building on the information learned during reintroduction. You will be introducing the foods you were able to tolerate regularly, and in combination with each other. Although I will provide some basic information to get you started, it won't be as structured as the processes you have completed so far. This phase of the low-FODMAP diet does not have a schedule, designated meal plan, or outlined challenges. You will be the one to decide how quickly you want to advance your awareness. Over time you will discover the thresholds that are unique to you and your body.

As we start this last chapter in your FODMAP journey, I hope you are content with how your body feels. However, be assured that all of us have good and bad days. Even if your symptoms improve with the low-FODMAP diet, you may benefit from some fine-tuning. So, before we talk about how to begin phase 3, let's walk through some additional treatments, therapies, and strategies for improving IBS that you may want to explore further.

ADDITIVE TREATMENTS

You may have been wondering about the therapies that will be discussed in this section. I consider them "additive treatments" for IBS. These include probiotics, cognitive behavioral therapy, fiber, enzymes, supplements, and other treatments designed to help alleviate IBS symptoms.

I did not recommend incorporating these treatments prior to this phase of the low-FODMAP diet, as they could impact your interpretation of the challenges. However, you have reached the point where you are free to explore their benefits.

The majority of the therapies that I describe in this section have shown modest results in alleviating symptoms for IBS patients. They may provide extra support to your gut health, used in conjunction with the low-FODMAP diet.

PROBIOTICS

Most of us have seen the advertisements or heard encouraging information about probiotics. While they won't be the "cure'" for IBS for most people, they can be helpful in controlling symptoms.

A probiotic is defined as a "live microorganism" (bacteria or yeast) that can offer health benefits when consumed in sufficient quantities. Probiotics typically exert their effects when they make their way to the intestines and help colonize the organ's microbiome (see "The Intestinal Microbiome," page 23). Therefore, it is crucial they survive the digestive activity of the mouth and stomach.

The organisms, or bacteria, that we know are most impacted by IBS and dietary modifications are lactobacillus, bifidobacterium, and bacillus. A recent meta-analysis suggested that among all probiotics, the ones containing lactobacillus present the strongest evidence for benefiting IBS patients. The authors endorsed taking the probiotics for a duration of four to eight weeks, but optimal timing was uncertain.

Probiotic labels will indicate which bacteria they contain and at what concentration (described as colony forming units, CFU). However, to date, there is no particular brand, or recommended CFU concentration, that should be ingested daily. Some probiotics can be kept at room temperature, and others require refrigeration.

A great resource to peruse available options is the *Clinical Guide to Probiotic Products Available in USA* (www.usprobioticguide.com). Select "Adult Health" from the drop-down menu to find their probiotic recommendations for IBS.

Popular products that have reliable manufacturing techniques include Align, Florastor, and Culturelle. Know that probiotics, like all over-the-counter supplements, are unregulated by the Federal Drug Administration (FDA).

I want to stress the importance of reading the ingredient list of your probiotics, as MANY products incorporate other high-FODMAP *prebiotic* ingredients such as inulin, which can worsen your symptoms.

COGNITIVE BEHAVIORAL THERAPY (CBT) OR HYPNOTHERAPY

Cognitive behavioral therapy is an intervention that typically involves a variety of techniques to change individual thinking patterns, improve coping skills, and increase confidence. The American Gastroenterological Association has endorsed considering psychological interventions for patients with moderate to severe IBS who do not respond to standard medical care, or for whom psychological factors exacerbate their symptoms.

Overall, there are few well-designed studies assessing this modality, but among the available information both CBT and gut-directed hypnotherapy may benefit those who did not respond to typical care.

SUPPLEMENTAL FIBER

We have all been told, at some point or another, that fiber is the key to helping our IBS woes. Indeed, for many years, this was the number one treatment doctors recommended, particularly for constipation symptoms. However, depending on the person and the type of fiber, we have since learned it may not be the answer. Not to mention, problems with bowel movements may have other causes, such as a pelvic floor disorder. (See "Prolapse and Problems with Poop," page 163, for more information about this common but underdiscussed issue.)

Fiber comes in many forms and has many properties. Soluble fiber (such as oats and psyllium) draws water into the colon and thus may be beneficial for treating constipation. Insoluble fiber (such as bran and corn) is not well digested, which can aid in bowel movement, but may irritate the gut.

The recommended daily fiber intake is 21 to 25 grams for women, and 30 to 38 grams for men. While many studies in the past decade have suggested that individuals on the low-FODMAP diet are at risk for low fiber consumption, the average American reportedly only consumes 12 to 18 grams each day.

I believe that it is quite possible to reach your recommended fiber allocation while following the low-FODMAP diet if you focus on low-FODMAP fiber sources. These include nuts and seeds, vegetables such as broccoli and potatoes, fruits such as kiwi and raspberries, and grains such as oats and quinoa.

The big question is, should you add *additional* fiber, through a supplement? The answer is, it depends.

In some cases, adding fiber to the diet can worsen symptoms, particularly at the beginning, if not started slowly. In other cases, it doesn't make enough difference to justify the cost and effort involved. Few studies have evaluated the use of fiber and the low-FODMAP diet together, and a good understanding of this dual therapy is lacking.

If you do decide you want to test this treatment, you have several choices. Psyllium (Metamucil), methylcellulose (Citrucel), calcium polycarbophil (FiberCon), wheat dextrin (Benefiber), and acacia fiber are commercially available and have been noted to benefit those with IBS (constipation and diarrhea). Similarly, partially hydrolyzed guar gum (PHGG) products have been FODMAP tested (Sunfiber and Regular Girl) and seem to work well in IBS-D.

If you do decide to pick an available option, be sure to drink plenty of water with your selection. Be cautious (as always) to read labels and avoid supplements that include irritants such as inulin, chicory root extract, and bran.

PROLAPSE AND PROBLEMS WITH POOP

Constipation is not the only reason people have problems pooping. There may be a structural barrier, or blockage, to the bowel movements. Possible causes are pelvic organ prolapse (rectocele, uterine prolapse, vaginal prolapse, and/or enterocele) and an inability to properly relax the muscles around the rectum (pelvic floor dyssynergia). These conditions lead to the sensation of incomplete emptying, straining, a need to push around the rectum to help defecate, and rectal pressure. Symptoms could begin any time, but often increase gradually. These disorders can occur in both women *and* men.

If you suspect you have one of these issues, then I recommend discussing it with your primary care provider. They may suggest a referral to a urogynecologist (like me!) or colorectal surgeon.

Beneficial treatments include pelvic floor physical therapy (yes, there are physical therapists who specialize in treating pelvic conditions), changing posture during defecation to improve stool passage (try putting your feet up on a stool in front of your commode or buy a "squatty potty"), and surgical options.

These problems are common and fixable, so don't be embarrassed to speak up.

ENZYMES

An alluring group of products, enzymes hold the promise of allowing us to keep eating the foods we enjoy *without adjustments*. Commercially available enzymes aid with the digestion of lactose, GOS, fructose, and inulin. While some have undergone FODMAP certification, few have been studied in IBS patients.

An enzyme is a protein made by our body to break down food, typically produced by the microbiome in our intestines. Synthetically produced enzymes replicate this action and thereby help digest the FODMAPs that create IBS flares. Here are a few of the common ones.

LACTASE

For those with lactose intolerance, research studies have proven that the lactase enzyme (sold commercially as products like Lactaid) is helpful in treating symptoms. Therefore, it is reasonable to use this as a supplemental tool to the low-FODMAP diet, if you want to consume a higher lactose meal than your tolerance allows. However, because most IBS patients have other FODMAP intolerances, this alone is not enough to treat all symptoms.

ALPHA-GALACTOSIDASE

Alpha-galactosidase is the enzyme that breaks down GOS. Intake of this enzyme has been studied in a small sample of patients with IBS. They found that for those on the low-FODMAP diet, using a full-strength dose of this enzyme (300 GALU) did facilitate tolerance of GOS-containing foods. Note that one of the familiar products for this, Beano, contains mannitol and thus isn't a low-FODMAP selection.

XYLOSE ISOMERASE

Xylose isomerase aids in fructose digestion. It has proven useful in treating fructose malabsorption, but studies are lacking in documenting its effectiveness in patients with IBS.

INULINASE

Inulinase is a component of a combination enzyme product designed to help with FODMAP digestion. The manufacturer claims this enzyme is helpful in breaking down fructans. Unfortunately, to date these claims have not been supported by published research.

MY BOTTOM LINE ON ENZYMES

Feel free to try an enzyme product as an occasional tool for use at a social gathering or other event where you can't be in control of the menu. It could improve your symptoms. However, I don't believe enzymes can replace following a modified low-FODMAP diet on a daily basis.

GLUTAMINE SUPPLEMENTATION

Glutamine is an amino acid supplement that is available over the counter in both powder and capsule forms. Glutamine has been demonstrated to help support the intestinal microbiome and thereby improve both constipation and diarrhea.

A recent study evaluated fifty people with IBS on the low-FODMAP diet who were supplemented with 15 grams of glutamine daily, compared with a similar group randomized to placebo. The authors reported improvement in IBS symptoms, stool consistency, stool frequency, and quality of life among those who took the glutamine.

Based on this research study, it appears reasonable to consider adding glutamine to your daily routine, if you are looking for some additional GI support. However, be aware that most supplements require three times daily dosing to reach the recommended intake, and cost could be a factor in maintaining this therapy.

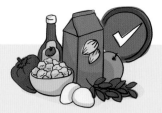

IT'S ALL ABOUT BALANCE

At the end of the day, a balanced diet is what we are striving for. Discovering which of the FODMAPs you can tolerate, and in what amounts, will help you accomplish this goal. Once you have established that information, you should aim to eat an array of fruits, vegetables, grains, and proteins each day. A varied menu provides the best nutritional balance, benefits your microbiome diversity, and allows for greater creativity.

The Healthy Eating Plate, as detailed by Harvard University's School of Nutrition, describes an "ideal" meal as 50 percent vegetables and fruits, 25 percent whole grains, and 25 percent protein sources. Oils should be used in moderation, avoiding partially hydrogenated options.

Here is one example of a balanced low-FODMAP plate:

- 1 cup (75 g) of steamed broccoli and carrots
- ½ cup (80 g) of baked potato, quinoa, or brown rice
- ¼ cup (60 g) of fish, chicken, or beef, cooked in olive or avocado oil

OPTIMIZE YOUR EATING STYLE

While not something most people think about, there may be an ideal eating style for minimizing IBS symptoms. Our intestines function in specific ways both during and between meals. Encouraging those functions helps control our gut balance and minimize flares.

Eating triggers an important physiological response called the *gastrocolic reflex*. This reflex varies in its intensity but occurs when a bolus of food interacts with our stomachs, causing neuropeptide and hormone secretion. The gastrocolic reflex helps propel food into the intestines and may lead to an urge to have a bowel movement shortly following a meal (often a good thing).

Not eating, or fasting between meals, stimulates intestinal "cleansing waves" known as *migrating motor complexes*. These waves help prepare the intestines for another meal and are of benefit to reducing accumulations in the gut (another good thing).

Thus, from a physiological standpoint, our intestines work best in a setting of regular, modest-sized meals, with 2- to 3-hour breaks in between.

Grazing is a practice where a person eats very small amounts of food in an unplanned manner throughout the day, but not necessarily when hungry. Grazing eliminates the body from establishing a pattern of mealtimes and reduces the cleansing intervals. As a result, optimal bowel functioning is impacted.

I suggest patients partake in three moderately sized meals a day and limit frequent snacking between. Avoid grazing when possible. Eating at relatively predictable times each day and eating food slowly has also been associated with reduced IBS symptoms in research studies.

WHAT ABOUT INTERMITTENT FASTING?

Intermittent fasting is an eating pattern that, while not new, has been increasing in popularity the last few years. Reasons for adopting it include weight loss and improving general health, among others.

I typically do not recommend "dieting" while *beginning* the low-FODMAP diet, as there are so many other challenges to the process. Nevertheless, as a lifelong plan, that may not be realistic.

However, there is no data evaluating the efficacy of fasting *in conjunction* with a modified low-FODMAP diet. The only research available on patients with IBS was a small study that compared symptoms in psychiatric patients who fasted for several consecutive days with those who did not. The group that fasted had greater improvements in abdominal pain, diarrhea, and bloating, but the study had several weaknesses. I don't think the findings can be generalized to represent results from intermittent fasting.

While there are different techniques for intermittent fasting, the practice often involves consuming a large "feast" of calories over a short period of the day. Consequently, there would be the potential to consume an excess of FODMAPs in a smaller interval of time. This load of FODMAPs may not be easily digested by a person with IBS. Furthermore, there is poor information on how fasting impacts the intestinal microbiome. Therefore, until further research in this area has been done, I suggest avoiding intermittent fasting while treating IBS with the low-FODMAP diet.

PUTTING IT ALL TOGETHER:
INTEGRATION AND PERSONALIZATION

By now, you should know which FODMAPs you tolerate, whether in small amounts or large portions. With that knowledge, you can start to enjoy foods that contain that FODMAP on a regular basis. If you completed the FODMAP combination challenges, you can incorporate that information into your eating plan as well.

As you navigate this new normal, gently add more variety to your menu. Begin by regularly combining two FODMAP categories at meals, then increase to a third. For example, you could try enjoying your yogurt topped with almonds and blackberries to test lactose, sorbitol, and GOS together.

There is no defined schedule for how this should happen. Each person is different regarding their preferred speed to advance their understanding. If you are someone who prefers structure, then feel free to be systematic about how you combine foods, and in what quantities. You may wish to continue break days in your regimen and maintain journaling. Do what feels good and right for you.

Remember that some ingredients contain a combination of more than two FODMAPs, and to always keep your eye on portion size. For example, tolerating the fructan challenge for garlic and the GOS challenge for chickpeas doesn't necessarily mean you can have hummus at a party. That hummus may have been made with dried and rehydrated chickpeas (not canned) and an abundance of garlic (much more than 4 grams per serving).

I recommend sticking to a balanced diet of whole foods at regular intervals. Eating at home is always my personal preference because I know my recipes are full of flavor and gentle on the tummy. Prepackaged and frozen foods contain additives and chemicals that challenge the digestion of people with IBS, whereas restaurant portions are often oversized and laden with hidden fats that can irritate the gut.

For me, while I eat nuts daily, I can't combine more than two vegetable and fruit portions in one sitting. If I have a smoothie, I use two of my favorite fruits, and if I make a vegetable stir-fry, I watch my serving size. I learned all of this through careful reintroduction testing, followed by a considered integration and personalization phase. While it sounds frustrating to be so aware of my food intake, I'm happy to be avoiding the abdominal bloating, lack of sleep, and low energy I experienced prior to discovering the low-FODMAP diet.

Eventually, you will fall into a pattern of knowing what you can and can't tolerate. Some people recognize they have few restrictions, while others, like me, are more sensitive. Regardless of your outcome, the knowledge you gain will empower your next steps.

Over time your tolerances and sensitivities could fluctuate. Changes to your health, medication adjustments, and modifications to your personal stressors could lead to more, or less, flexibility in your diet. I always tell my patients that medicine is unpredictable. There is so much that we don't know or understand. You may wish to try certain FODMAP challenges again in a few weeks or months to see if you have a different outcome.

For now, my advice is to embrace this stage of your low-FODMAP lifestyle. You are benefiting from a more varied and flexible menu: your personalized low-FODMAP diet. It will look different than mine, as it should. We have unique bodies and individual needs.

I am so glad to have you join me here, on this side of the low-FODMAP diet: free of IBS symptoms and enjoying a balanced, healthy eating plan.

Cheers to our digestive wellness.

Forever.

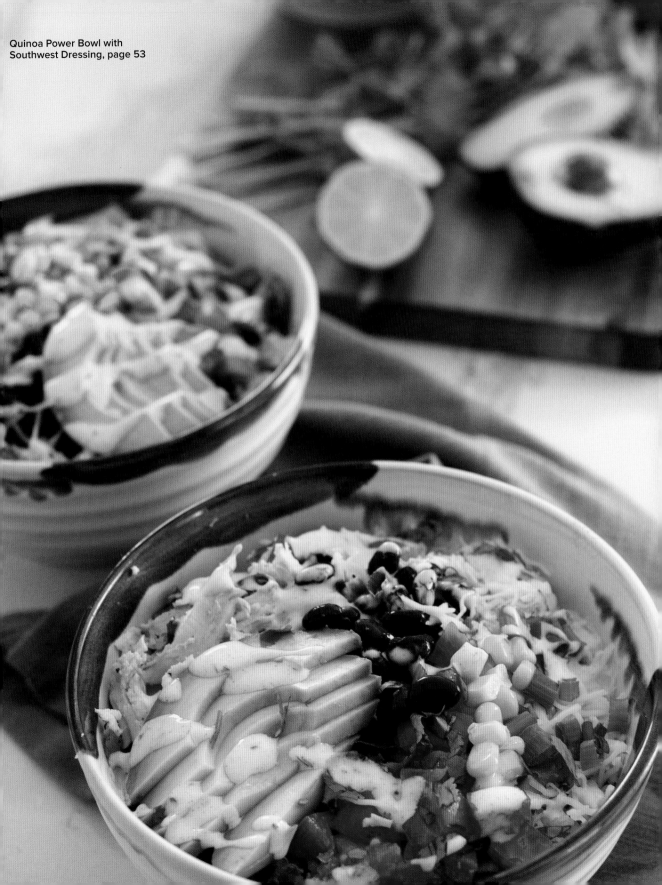

Quinoa Power Bowl with
Southwest Dressing, page 53

REFERENCES

Black, C. J., E. R. Thakur, L. A. Houghton, E. M. M. Quigley, P. Moayyedi, and A. C. Ford. 2020. Efficacy of psychological therapies for irritable bowel syndrome: Systematic review and network meta-analysis. *Gut* 69 (8): 1441–1451.

Chey, W. D., J. G. Hashash, L. Manning, and L. Chang. 2022. AGA clinical practice update on the role of diet in irritable bowel syndrome: Expert review. *Gastroenterology* 162 (6): 1737–1745.

Harvie, R. M., A. W. Chisholm, J. E. Bisanz, J. P. Burton, P. Herbison, K. Schultz, and M. Schultz. 2017. Long-term irritable bowel syndrome symptom control with reintroduction of selected FODMAPs. *World Journal of Gastroenterology* 23 (25): 4632–4643.

Lacy, B. E., M. Pimentel, D. M. Brenner, W. D. Chey, L. A. Keefer, M. D. Long, and B. Moshiree. 2021. ACG clinical guideline: Management of irritable bowel syndrome. *American Journal of Gastroenterology* 116 (1): 17–44.

Liu, J., W. D. Chey, E. Haller, and S. Eswaran. 2020. Low-FODMAP diet for irritable bowel syndrome: What we know and what we have yet to learn. *Annual Review of Medicine* 71: 303–314.

Rastgoo, S., N. Ebrahimi-Daryani, S. Agah, S. Karimi, M. Taher, B. Rashidkhani, E. Hejazi, F. Mohseni, M. Ahmadzadeh, A. Sadeghi, and A. Hekmatdoost. 2021. Glutamine supplementation enhances the effects of a low FODMAP diet in irritable bowel syndrome management. *Frontiers in Nutrition* 8: 746703.

So, D., C. K. Yao, Z. S. Ardalan, P. A. Thwaites, K. Kalantar-Zadeh, P. R. Gibson, and J. G. Muir. 2021. Supplementing dietary fibers with a low FODMAP diet in irritable bowel syndrome: A randomized controlled crossover trial. *Clinical Gastroenterology and Hepatology* 18: S1542.

Tuck, C., and J. Barrett. 2017. Re-challenging FODMAPs: The low FODMAP diet phase two. *Journal of Gastroenterology and Hepatology* 32 (Suppl 1): 11–15.

Whelan, K., L. D. Martin, H. M. Staudacher, and M. C. E. Lomer. 2018. The low FODMAP diet in the management of irritable bowel syndrome: An evidence-based review of FODMAP restriction, reintroduction and personalisation in clinical practice. *Journal of Human Nutrition and Dietetics* 31 (2): 239–255.

Xie, C. R., B. Tang, Y. Z. Shi, W. Y. Peng, K. Ye, Q. F. Tao, S. G. Yu, H. Zheng, and M. Chen. 2020. Low FODMAP diet and probiotics in irritable bowel syndrome: A systematic review with network meta-analysis. *Frontiers in Pharmacology* 13: 853011.

RESOURCES

MONASH UNIVERSITY

Originators of a large volume of low-FODMAP research and creators of the Monash University FODMAP Diet app.

www.monashfodmap.com

FODMAP FRIENDLY

Reliable resource for FODMAP testing data and creators of the FODMAP Friendly app.

www.fodmapfriendly.com

INTERNATIONAL FOUNDATION FOR GASTROINTESTINAL DISORDERS

A nonprofit education and research organization with information about IBS.

www.aboutibs.org

RACHEL PAULS FOOD (MY WEBSITE)

Informative blog with medical information and more than 500 free low-FODMAP recipes and source for delicious laboratory-certified low-FODMAP food products, including energy bars (Happy Bars), soup bases (Happy Soup), spice blends (Happy Spices), and baking mixes (Happy Baking).

www.rachelpaulsfood.com

FODMAP EVERYDAY

Useful blogs and recipes for the low-FODMAP diet.

www.fodmapeveryday.com

PATSY CATSOS, MS, RDN

Patsy is an expert gastroenterology dietitian and book author.

www.ibsfree.net

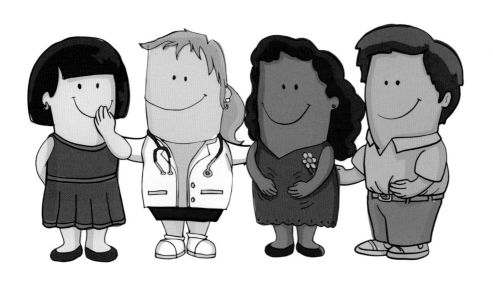

ACKNOWLEDGMENTS

This book would not have been possible without the following individuals:

My husband, Cory: You are my backbone and partner in every way. Thank you for your support, your friendship, and your love.

My children, Hannah, Jack, and Zev: My greatest accomplishment, you inspire all I do. I can't wait to see what each stage of your lives brings.

My mother and friend, Jeanne: A co-cooking enthusiast and best FODMAP recipe tester ever. Your input for this book was invaluable and will be cherished always.

Drs. Catrina and Jennifer: Like sisters, our bond is deep, honest, and real. You are both incredibly special and talented people.

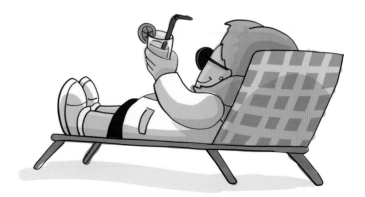

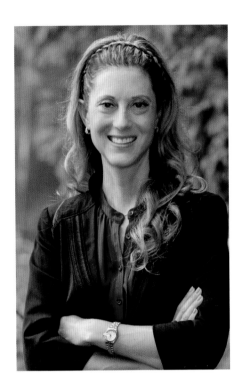

ABOUT THE AUTHOR

Dr. Rachel Pauls is an internationally renowned surgeon and medical researcher who is also a passionate chef and FODMAP blogger. She has published more than one hundred original medical journal articles and book chapters and served as the program director for the Fellowship Program in Female Pelvic Medicine and Reconstructive Surgery for nine years, and director of research for the Division of Urogynecology at TriHealth in Cincinnati, Ohio, for twelve years. She is currently a busy clinician, pelvic surgeon, and mother of three.

An IBS sufferer, Dr. Pauls follows a modified low-FODMAP diet to successfully eliminate her own symptoms. In order to help others solve their digestive issues, Dr. Pauls founded Rachel Pauls Food, one of the world's leading makers of delicious laboratory-certified low-FODMAP food, in 2016. Her website, www.rachelpaulsfood.com, has more than 500 low-FODMAP recipes and a line of delicious low-FODMAP food products such as energy bars (Happy Bars), soup bases (Happy Soup), spice blends (Happy Spices), and baking mixes (Happy Baking). Her acclaimed first book, *The Low-FODMAP IBS Solution Plan and Cookbook*, was published in 2020.

INDEX